T0269275

Planning for a Career in Biomedical and Life Sciences

Planning for a Career in Biomedical and Life Sciences

Learn to Navigate a Tough Research Culture by Harnessing the Power of Career Building

Second Edition

Avrum I. Gotlieb MDCM, FRCPC
Professor, Department of Laboratory Medicine and Pathobiology
Faculty of Medicine, University of Toronto
Toronto, ON, Canada

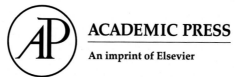

ACADEMIC PRESS
An imprint of Elsevier

Academic Press is an imprint of Elsevier
125 London Wall, London EC2Y 5AS, United Kingdom
525 B Street, Suite 1650, San Diego, CA 92101-4495, United States
50 Hampshire Street, 5th Floor, Cambridge, MA 02139, United States
The Boulevard, Langford Lane, Kidlington, Oxford OX5 1GB, United Kingdom

Notices
Knowledge and best practice in this field are constantly changing. As new research and experience broaden our
understanding, changes in research methods, professional practices, or medical treatment may become
necessary.

Practitioners and researchers must always rely on their own experience and knowledge in evaluating and using
any information, methods, compounds, or experiments described herein. In using such information or methods
they should be mindful of their own safety and the safety of others, including parties for whom they have a
professional responsibility.

To the fullest extent of the law, neither the Publisher nor the authors, contributors, or editors, assume any
liability for any injury and/or damage to persons or property as a matter of products liability, negligence or
otherwise, or from any use or operation of any methods, products, instructions, or ideas contained in the
material herein.

British Library Cataloguing-in-Publication Data
A catalogue record for this book is available from the British Library

Library of Congress Cataloging-in-Publication Data
A catalog record for this book is available from the Library of Congress

ISBN: 978-0-12-814978-2

For Information on all Academic Press publications
visit our website at https://www.elsevier.com/books-and-journals

  Working together
to grow libraries in
developing countries

www.elsevier.com • www.bookaid.org

Publisher: Mica Haley
Acquisition Editor: Mary Preap
Editorial Project Manager: Mary Preap
Production Project Manager: Punithavathy Govindaradjane
Cover Designer: Miles Hitchen

Typeset by MPS Limited, Chennai, India

DEDICATION

Dedicated to my wife, Linda and to the memory of my parents, Harry and Roberta Gotlieb.

CONTENTS

**Hard Work, Self-Reflection, Resilience and New Knowledge
Go Hand in Hand in Career Development**

Independence in a Protected Environment

Life Continues But the Rules Are Different

**Your Initial Employment Is Still Part of the Journey
and Not Your Destination**

**Teaching and Research Institutions Are Valuable Community Resources
and Require Constant Care**

ABOUT THE AUTHOR

I have a long-time passion for postsecondary education in life sciences and biomedical research. I am the founding Chair of the Department of Laboratory Medicine and Pathobiology (LMP), Faculty of Medicine, University of Toronto (1997–2008). Following my Chairmanship, I was Interim Vice Dean, Research and International Relations (2009–10) and Acting and Interim Vice Dean, Graduate 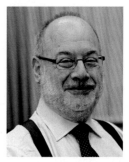 and Life Sciences Education (2011–14) in the Faculty of Medicine. I was Senior Academic Advisor to the Dean, Faculty of Medicine, University of Toronto (2010–17).

I received BSc in Psychology and Physiology, with first class honors (1967), and MDCM (1971) from McGill University. I continued my training in medicine and anatomic pathology at the teaching hospitals of McGill University. I received fellowship from the Royal College of Physicians and Surgeons of Canada in Anatomic Pathology (1975) and certification from the American Board of Pathology (1976). I pursued research training in cell biology in the Department of Biology, University of California San Diego with Professor S.J. Singer, supported by a Medical Research Council Fellowship.

My interest in career planning began as Course Director of the new Pathobiology course in Undergraduate Medicine, which was part of a then new curriculum for medical students. To meet the career development needs of these groups of students, I wrote my first career development booklet in 2003, which is now in its 4th edition "The Road to Becoming a Biomedical Physician Scientist in Pathology and Laboratory Medicine," published by the American Society for Investigative Pathology, Bethesda, MD with support from the Intersociety Council for Pathology Information.

I had two other leadership positions as Coordinator of Graduate Studies in Pathology, which trained primarily nonclinical students and two decades ago, I planned and initiated with colleagues an educational program that was an innovative and unique undergraduate arts and science Specialist Program in Pathobiology. The goal was to introduce non-MDs very early on in their life science training to the research world of mechanisms of disease. As I worked with these graduate and undergraduate students, I began to realize how poorly prepared they were to plan their own careers. To fill the gap, I wrote and published "Planning a Career in Biomedical and Life Sciences: Making Informed Choices."

My own research interests include atherosclerosis and valvular heart disease. I have published on blood vessel repair, especially on the role of the cytoskeleton in endothelial repair, and I also studied how heart valve cells repair valves after they have been injured. I authored over 100 peer-reviewed papers, and 35 reviews and book chapters. I edited three books, including the comprehensive textbook Cardiovascular Pathology, edited with colleagues M.D. Silver, University of Toronto, and F. Schoen, Harvard Medical School. I have received peer-reviewed funding from the Heart and Stroke Foundation of Ontario and the Medical Research Council, now Canadian Institutes of Health Research (CIHR).

I found the task around publishing scientific and clinical studies very rewarding. I am the past coeditor of Cardiovascular Pathology, a journal of the Society for Cardiovascular Pathology dedicated to basic, clinical, and applied cardiovascular science published by Elsevier. I serve in the Editorial Board of The American Journal of Pathology (AJP) and of Laboratory Investigation. I am an associate editor of Cardiovascular Pathology and a senior advisor, Academic Pathology.

I have enjoyed serving the scientific and medical community in a variety of ways to provide leadership, advocacy, and to help maintain high quality scholarship for students and faculty. I am a former President of the American Society for Investigative Pathology (ASIP) and past President of the Canadian Society of Atherosclerosis, Thrombosis and Vascular Biology (CSATVB), and the Society for Cardiovascular Pathology (SCVP). I was a member of the Board of the Federation of American Societies of Experimental Biology (FASEB) and served as FASEB Vice President for Science Policy. I am an elected Fellow of the Canadian Academy of Health Sciences and a Senior Fellow of the Association of Pathology Chairs.

I was honored to be recognized by the SCVP with the Distinguished Achievement Award, by the ASIP with the Robbins Distinguished Educator Award, by the Association of Pathology Chairs with their Distinguished Service Award, and by the Canadian Association of Pathologists with the President's Award. I have presented career talks at several national and international scientific meetings and venues and consider mentorship, education, and career development as the highlights of my own career.

Despite emerging local curricula, the availability of much online information, and numerous other sources that focus on specific aspects of career planning, you need a comprehensive narrative to guide you to be resilient and embrace your task of career planning. This book pulls together the experiences of a successful biomedical researcher and academic leader and validates the diverse scattered information available on social media to create an authoritative narrative. As you navigate the unpredictable waters of life sciences and biomedical research, it is sink or swim. You need to know what to expect and how to handle the challenges so that you can thrive in a tough research culture that is very demanding of time and effort and requires rigorous intellectual focus. Reading the book in sequence will provide you with an appreciation of how to become part of the culture and community of life sciences research and how to plan strategically at each stage of your career. Even early on, it is useful to know mid-range and long-range issues even though you are dealing with the short term and focusing on short-term deliverables. It is important to read the full narrative. This makes strategic planning much more effective. Students and faculty who have done this with the first edition found it very rewarding. After a full reading of the book, you will be able to harness the power of planning and reread specific issues as they come up in your planning, for example, how to choose your mentors, how to choose a graduate program, and how to prepare for job interviews.

Preparing for a career in life sciences and biomedical research is a daunting task which requires comprehensive and accurate information on what to expect, how to plan, how to avoid pitfalls, and how to be resilient and enjoy the journey to success. The main tenet of this book is that career planning requires accurate information about this complex world of academic and nonacademic life sciences and biomedical research. The objective of my efforts is to provide you as students and junior faculty a competitive advantage by presenting a practical guide with useful information, insights, and tips to guide you on your journey of career planning as you achieve milestones and competencies in your biomedical and life sciences professions.

The book focuses on how best to make plans for a successful career and urges you to begin by carrying out self-reflection to understand how well a research career in life sciences, whether in the academic or industrial world, fits you. These dynamic plans, if carried out well, provide the opportunity to make informed choices during training, job searching, and job performance in the very competitive academic and nonacademic job market. This focus on both sectors is important since these are both very competitive job markets for life sciences graduates. Much has been written on career development; but, with the dramatic increase in career choices available for biomedical and life sciences research graduates, students and faculty need a comprehensive approach to meet the challenges of preparing for the job market. In this job market, careers do not just develop spontaneously; to have a fair shot at success, planning and dynamic strategies are crucial. Students have to be aggressive and devote time and energy creating their own career plans. In the final analysis, it is up to you to chart your own course by using resources such as this book and turning to devoted people and mentors along the way.

Due to major scientific and social disruptions, there is clearly a global call for strategic career planning to ensure that training dollars are well spent and young scientists are successfully trained to compete for highly skilled competitive research and research-associated jobs. You are overwhelmed by disruptive and transformative changes, faculty are trying desperately to understand and perform in this changing job market/environment, and employers are often expressing frustration with a work force that is lacking in skills for success. Science leadership, faculty, students, and employers are looking for strategies to effectively use dynamic planning in career development for the benefit of the biomedical and life sciences research communities. You, as a student, should use this book to plan ahead and set clear milestones to achieve competencies required by the job market.

It is over 3 years since I completed the manuscript for the first edition of my book "Planning a Career in Biomedical and Life Sciences: Making Informed Choices." Even in this short period of time, the area of career development in life sciences has evolved greatly. Career development has become a serious issue at NIH and at other funding agencies and is being scrutinized as part of grant applications for research funding. More scholarly papers have been written about career planning lately. Career development is slowly entering the curriculum of some academic programs that train students in biomedical and life sciences research. This new curriculum is often referred to as Graduate Professional Development by graduate training programs.

As an academic leader, I hope that this book will be used by faculty mentors and supervisors who interact with trainees and junior faculty to help prepare students for a successful career in a job market that has changed significantly since their own youth. These mentors and supervisors have a considerable role to play in guiding their protégés during the most defining years of their lives. This book provides information to help supervisors understand the needs of today's students that reflect the scientific communities we live in. Several colleagues who read the first edition of this book told me that they wish they had a book like this when they were training and launching their own careers.

I would like to acknowledge valuable interviews and discussions with numerous colleagues, both in the academic and nonacademic communities, trainees, and students who shared their thoughts with me on career planning. Their views on academic training and scholarship, on mentorship, and on the value of student extracurricular activities are much appreciated. I thank those students and faculty whom I personally mentored for their useful feedback especially on health and wellness, resilience, and work–life balance. It is clear to me that our current students face a different world than my colleagues and I faced when we were planning and launching our own careers. As supervisors and mentors, we must understand the changes and help prepare you, our students, for successful careers.

I would like to thank my own mentors who were willing to devote time and energy to help me shape my own career and those of many of my colleagues as we progressed through our education and career planning. These mentors helped me to make informed choices along the journey of my own career development. For this I am eternally grateful.

I appreciate the input of Professors Michelle Bendeck and Jeffrey Lee, Department of Laboratory Medicine and Pathobiology,

University of Toronto, and the assistance of Bessie Gorospe, Graduate and Life Sciences Education, Faculty of Medicine, and Heather Seto, Joanne D'Angelo and Maria Tinajero Laboratory Medicine and Pathobiology, University of Toronto. I appreciate the helpful comments and discussions on nonacademic careers in life sciences with Songyi Xu, a graduate student in Laboratory Medicine and Pathobiology and formerly Co-President of the Life Sciences Career Development Society, University of Toronto. I am grateful to Meshulam Gotlieb for his continued professionalism and imagination in helping me develop and further clarify important aspects of both the first and second editions of the book. His wonderful ideas and helpful comments especially concerning resilience and mindfulness contributed significantly to the overall tone and style of the text.

Avrum I. Gotlieb
January 2018

Inspiration and Passion Are Useful Companions on Your Journey

CHAPTER 1

Inspired by Life Sciences

1.1 HIGH SCHOOL—A PLACE TO BE INSPIRED
1.2 LIFESTYLE IN THE BIOSCIENCE COMMUNITY

SUMMARY

You may have developed a passion early on for the life sciences and thus you wish to explore a career in this field, even as early as high school. Dream big and work hard to make these dreams a reality. As a prospective life science student, seek information about the life science and biomedical research community to understand how you may fit into various life science careers. Your goal is to align your career goals and your strengths and weaknesses with the requirements and demands of various life sciences careers. Your initial consideration is selecting appropriate educational opportunities, the first of which is your under-graduate institution and program. Take time to speak with high school guidance counselors. Search for current information on the Internet. Visit college/university information fairs. You should ensure that your information on entrance requirements, programs, and scholarships is up to date since requirements and deadlines do frequently change. Identify any barriers that may prevent you from obtaining postsecondary educa-tion. Learn how to overcome barriers through contact with guidance councillors, teachers, and others, some of whom may have successfully navigated their own barriers. Find out about pipeline and outreach pro-grams that will help you gain insight into university life. These are very useful to underrepresented and low-income communities. Contact with mentors helps guide you in making informed short-term and long-term career plans. The lifestyle in life sciences is highly desirable as it allows you to be immersed in a fast-paced and ever changing environment. It is hard work but it is also fun and exciting. You join the global commu-nity of like-minded scientists who expand the knowledge base and the applications of biomedical and life science.

Planning for a Career in Biomedical and Life Sciences. DOI: https://doi.org/10.1016/B978-0-12-814978-2.00001-6

1.1 HIGH SCHOOL—A PLACE TO BE INSPIRED

So why are you interested in biomedical and life sciences research? Does your interest date back to high school or even earlier? Are you curious to know how living organisms work? Was your interest piqued by the complex world surrounding you, or were you inspired by a mentor, a relative, or a friend? Was your early interest channeled by TV shows, movies, the Internet, teachers, or field trips that opened your mind to the questions posed by biology, and informed you of the opportunities available to solve the riddles of the biosciences.

You probably began studying biology in the form of lectures and assignments on how the cells and the molecules inside and outside the cell control human biology. Internet life science sites probably further exposed you to the many fascinating stories of how tissues, cells, and molecules organize the many functions of micro-organisms, insects, animals, and humans. You may have been inspired by the videos of three-dimensional molecules that you were able to manipulate with your keyboard and by films of live cells moving and growing.

Biology is All Around Us

As you came to realize that life and biomedical sciences provide you with the keys to unlock and discover the workings of the human body, you may have been bitten by the bug to understand the molecular mysteries of the human organism! You may have been further inspired by visits from life sciences university students or professors to your high school. Their excitement about their own or others' new discoveries—that change how we think about biology, health, and disease—may have been contagious. If a member of your immediate family became seriously ill, you may have been motivated to harness science to prevent or cure the abnormal biology that leads to disease and human suffering.

Perhaps, during your high school years, you were coached by your science teacher when you participated in a science fair, or you even had the opportunity to carry out hands-on research in a real laboratory. As you move forward, do not forget to acknowledge those teachers who helped you early on. They like to hear how you are doing in university and beyond. They all fueled your initial interest.

To further pursue your interest, you may have attended research exhibits and university information fairs to obtain career information. On my own campus, information days for local high school students are well attended. Our program directors and students field questions all day long and information brochures rapidly disappear from our information booths. Students are interested in what the research opportunities are, while parents are more interested in job opportunities and the cost of education.

In high school, you should be provided with educational resources that foster your interest in attending college/university. You should have the opportunity to explore the benefits and challenges of higher education and come to believe that it is a realistic option for you. This is especially important if you are a student who comes from backgrounds that traditionally did not have the opportunities to attend college/university. Your family members may not have had the opportunities and/or the financial means to pursue postsecondary education. Career counselors are supposed to possess the up-to-date information that will enable you to enroll in postsecondary education. You should seek out programs available at the local, provincial, and federal level that have been successful in expanding opportunities for teenagers to help them prepare for and access postsecondary education.

These outreach programs are usually provided by individual schools, boards of education, and government agencies. Many colleges and universities also offer programs directed at less advantaged students to provide them with an opportunity to meet with active faculty and to attend and participate in lectures, seminars, and laboratory experiences. These offer a glimpse of what the future may hold for you. They provide you with the opportunity to make contact with potential mentors and figure out what you need to plan for. If you enjoy the pursuit of new knowledge and are excited by new discoveries, life sciences may be the career to satisfy these passions. The next step then is to begin to plan your career. Do not forget to dream big!

> Reach Out to Identify Opportunities

1.2 LIFESTYLE IN THE BIOSCIENCE COMMUNITY

Before you begin to plan in earnest, it pays to think about the lifestyle you are getting into. Is it right for you? You will be in a very fast moving and extremely competitive environment, whether you choose to be employed in the academy or in industry. You will find yourself working in a culture that values discovery and innovation. I can testify that I find myself surrounded by highly intelligent colleagues and extremely bright students. In addition to science, many of my colleagues and students are also immersed in life-enriching pursuits in music, art, and literature. This is a very exciting environment to be in. Research challenges are constantly being discussed and novel experiments described as you and your colleagues try to solve biologic and medical problems. Discussions are energized and stimulating and the ideas flow freely. Conversations always spill over into local and world issues. We have stimulating discussions on politics, religion, health care, poverty, and the income gap, to name a few. We also discuss the arts, the latest play in town, the newest film and, of course, sports. Although I live in a hockey city, baseball, basketball, and football catch our interest as well. Intense debates have occurred about soccer, especially during World Cup time. These lifestyle perks can be fun and certainly help create a collegial community. Furthermore, they integrate scientific research with the world at large.

Although the work is hard and quite time- and energy-consuming, you will have the opportunity to travel to present your research findings to colleagues at universities, research institutions, and scientific meetings. Science is an international endeavor, so you will develop a transglobal group of like-minded friends and acquaintances with whom you will share stimulating scientific and social experiences. You will get to see the world and interact with the international scientific community. For many of my colleagues this is worth the trials and tribulations of life sciences research. The journey through life sciences is fun and rewarding and does provide you with a fine work—life balance.

What can you look forward to? Choosing a career in life sciences commits you to lifelong learning even once you have settled into a job. Your knowledge will propel you outside the life sciences sphere into the community. You may have the opportunity to become a spokesperson or advocate extolling the value of the life sciences and

> Life Sciences Offers An Exciting Lifestyle

biomedical research to funders, politicians, and the lay public. You can provide guidance and leadership to many civic causes that will benefit greatly from your unique fund of knowledge, especially in public outreach forums. A career in biomedical and life sciences is more than a job: it is a lifestyle, an exciting and challenging one.

As a life scientist, you have been well educated. You are at the forefront of the knowledge and innovations economy. Society's investment in your education and your research brings with it many benefits, including advances in health, improved quality of life, job creation, and economic growth. You are at the forefront of biology. Your training provides you with unique insight into the many biological and biomedical events that you come across in daily life. You are trained to recognize disease conditions. You are able to understand the functions of your own body and how environmental agents may cause injury or disease. You have a better understanding than most people of disease and of how lifestyles can be either beneficial or harmful to the body. Likewise you can understand the effects of proper nutrition better than your neighbors. Life scientists are continuously exposed to new ideas and concepts as well as new techniques and technologies. Being a lifelong learner is an essential ingredient for success and also provides you with a contemporary knowledge base for civic engagement. I have found that my training in life sciences has been very helpful on so many levels, including carrying out my own professional duties as a pathologist and a laboratory physician.

Career Success Favors the Informed and Prepared Mind

CHAPTER 2

Your Dynamic Training Path

2.1 PUTTING YOUR BEST FOOT FORWARD
2.2 EARLY GUIDANCE
2.3 CHARTING PATHWAYS TO SUCCESS

SUMMARY

After serious self-reflection and self-assessment of your goals and your own strengths and weaknesses, collect information about careers in life sciences. You must now develop a written plan to identify pathways to achieve your career goals. This typically involves a combination of short- and long-range planning and includes identifying your educational goals and the competencies you need in order to achieve them. To help with this, identify and adhere to timelines and milestones. It is important to understand that your plans are most likely to change as interests and opportunities change; therefore, plans will need to be revised and modified often. It is also essential for you to recognize an opportunity when it suddenly appears. Give serendipity a chance. Furthermore, it is essential that the plan be flexible in case unforeseen disruptions occur, many of which you have no control over. Remaining well informed of your options will assist you greatly in revising your plan. Remember that you are living in a rapidly changing world where innovation, transformation, and disruption must be recognized and embraced as you plan your career. Consider gap years and time-outs during your education when you feel these will benefit your career planning.

2.1 PUTTING YOUR BEST FOOT FORWARD

To create or recreate a dynamic training path at any stage of your career, you need to step back and consider your own "life-career" paradigm in a thorough and honest way (Fig. 2.1). Self-knowledge and reflection, (the "who am I scenario"), and understanding the specific features of a specific career that you are considering will help you to

Planning for a Career in Biomedical and Life Sciences. DOI: https://doi.org/10.1016/B978-0-12-814978-2.00002-8

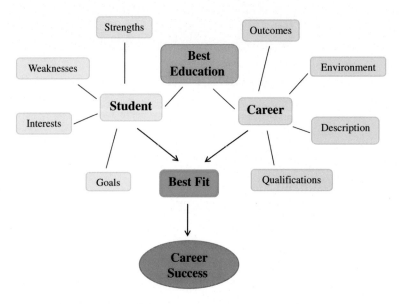

Figure 2.1 Designing a dynamic career plan.

achieve the best fit. The template included here, designing a dynamic career plan, is meant to provide you with the guidance necessary to keep yourself strategically focused. You may begin considering these issues in your early undergraduate years and make alterations and changes as you progress into graduate school and beyond. You need to start from somewhere and this is your initial plan. You need to be strategic to move your plan forward, but even more importantly, you need to pay constant attention as you enjoy the journey and recognize opportunities as they suddenly arise.

> Explore Your Own
> Life-Career Paradigm

I frequently hear the following remarks from both students and colleagues: "If only I would have known," "I missed the deadline to apply," and "If only someone would have told me to do this at the time, my career path would have been much smoother." If you spend the time and energy necessary to gather information on career development, these gripes can be avoided. You need to seek both general information that is relevant to most careers, such as writing a proper CV, and learning optimum interview techniques, and specific information relevant to your own areas of interest, such as the best schools to train at and the best journals to read. To your surprise, you will find information on topics you did not consider important to be crucial to your planning. By being attentive, you will slowly find many pieces to the puzzle that you might have otherwise overlooked because it never even occurred to you to search for them in the first place. Thus, to be successful, begin to immerse yourself early in career development, so that you are able to think ahead, plan ahead, and seize opportunities as they appear.

2.2 EARLY GUIDANCE

Life sciences is a broad topic, and deciding how to enter the area may be initially bewildering. It is up to you to actively seek out information. Do not be shy. Be polite but be persistent in obtaining the answers you need. Knowledgeable career counseling, especially from high school and university counselors and undergraduate and graduate program leaders, will help you learn what programs are available and what prerequisites and eligibility criteria exist. You should already be seeking guidance when you are still in high school. Guidance is just that. It does not commit you to a particular course of action; however, it provides you with valuable information and allows you to make informed choices. You need to keep information current because entrance requirements, programs, and scholarship opportunities do change. Make sure you have current and correct forms when filling out applications. The path you choose begins in high school, continues in undergraduate university, and leads into graduate and/or professional schools (Fig. 2.2). Following these phases, there is further postgraduate and postprofessional training. You may enter or leave the path at any stage. Peoples' interests and career plans often change. The inner forces that motivate students are the passion for what they are learning, the fun they have at work, and the societal and personal value apparent in their research.

> Make Informed Choices

> Have Fun and
> See the Value of Your Work

2.3 CHARTING PATHWAYS TO SUCCESS

A well thought-out training path will enable you to reach your career goals. Sometimes, however, you may choose to change in midcourse. One student I know had been moving in a certain direction for several years and was succeeding in this path. Between semesters, she took the opportunity to volunteer for an international placement in a third-

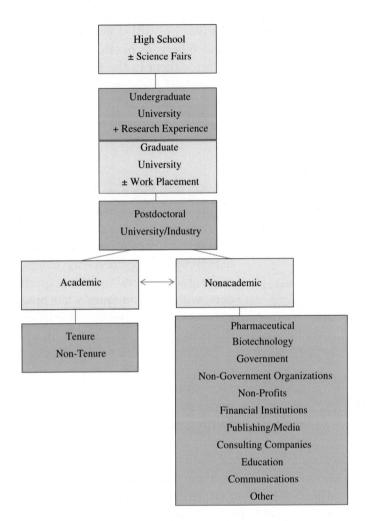

Figure 2.2 A traditional pathway.

world country. This experience opened her eyes to new career opportunities that she did not know even existed. Upon return, she discussed her experience with her mentors, carefully gathered as much relevant information as possible, and after weighing the pros and cons, altered her course of study to provide her with the expertise to follow her newly found passion.

Usually your career planning will combine short- and long-range components that combine to result in a carefully crafted individual development plan. You should begin by focusing on acquiring extremely high-quality training in a timely fashion. Some students thrive in programs that offer considerable flexibility, while others do well in more structured programs. However, no matter how well your plan is going, you must also be able to consider taking advantage of opportunities

> Consider Short and Long Range Planning

that appear unexpectedly as you follow your training plan. Serendipity may provide you with an outstanding opportunity. It may, however, take you off your path, thus demanding that you make an unexpected and difficult choice. In such a case, treat your plan as dynamic and subject to change, and carefully discuss the pros and cons of this opportunity with your mentors. Do not act on a whim, but be flexible. Even if nothing unexpected occurs, remember to revisit your plan at least every six months.

There is more than one way to reach your goal, so make sure to take your own personal circumstances into account when planning

> Planning and Serendipity

each step. Remember that although the outcome is important, the journey must be pleasant, fun, and as direct as possible so that you do not fall into the trap of becoming a perpetual trainee. Your objective should be to carefully establish deliberate career plans that are sufficiently flexible to respond to chance opportunities that appear from time to time.

Training paths in life sciences may be straight forward and traditional or circuitous and less traditional. The traditional path is high school biology followed by undergraduate studies with an emphasis in life sciences. This undergraduate period will also include laboratory research experience, which may take place in the guise of laboratory courses and research course projects. Experiential learning such as internships and work placements are also valuable experiences that may take place during this time. This phase is followed by graduate school and postdoctoral training. By the end of this path, you will be well prepared to take on an academic or a nonacademic job.

Alternatively, career pathways may be circuitous and include interruptions. You may step out of university and work for a while. This will provide income to support future studies and a change of environment, so that you may gain a better perspective on how you want your career to develop. Such a time-out is not uncommon. Some time-outs from formal education still keep you in a research laboratory environment as a technician. Others may find you travelling and seeing the world. During your travels you may choose to explore international study opportunities outside your own country that might appeal to you at a later date.

> Consider Educational Time-Outs in Your Career Plan

Dream Big and Settle for the Best You Can Accomplish

CHAPTER 3

Your Undergraduate Studies

3.1 CHOOSING YOUR UNDERGRADUATE EDUCATION
3.2 THE VALUE OF DEPTH VS BREADTH IN YOUR UNDERGRADUATE CURRICULUM
3.3 GUIDANCE IN SUCCESSFUL CAREER DEVELOPMENT
3.4 THE VALUE OF A MENTOR
3.5 HOW TO BEHAVE AS A MENTEE
3.6 ACHIEVING VALUE IN YOUR UNDERGRADUATE MENTORED RESEARCH OPPORTUNITY
3.7 MAKING THE MOST OF YOUR RESEARCH EXPERIENCE

SUMMARY

You will be exposed to two paths during your undergraduate education. One focuses on breadth training and the other on in-depth training. A combination or blending of the two is desirable as you will then experience both in-depth knowledge in a particular area and superficial knowledge in other areas. Specialist or honors programs focus on in-depth research and education. These allow you to embrace complex problems and demonstrate the strategies you use to solve them. Potential graduate supervisors will discuss these with you to assess your research potential. During undergraduate studies, it is critical that you gain hands-on undergraduate research experience to be considered for admission to graduate life science programs. Mentored undergraduate research opportunities should be embraced since engaging in research will provide you with the opportunity to learn first-hand how you might fit into the role of a graduate student in a life science biomedical laboratory. You will learn that you need to work hard and that you are likely to encounter successes and failures. Aside from family, friends, and partners, you are strongly advised to seek out suitable mentors early on for guidance and support. Mentorship is essential for successful career development. Mentorship should be a two-way street in which the mentee and the mentor have specific requirements and expectations. Each

Planning for a Career in Biomedical and Life Sciences. DOI: https://doi.org/10.1016/B978-0-12-814978-2.00003-X

will gain from this unique faculty–student relationship. To keep you on track, record an Undergraduate Diary to remind you of the competencies and milestones you will need to achieve along the early stages of your career path.

3.1 CHOOSING YOUR UNDERGRADUATE EDUCATION

You need to be well informed about the life sciences/biomedical sciences program offered at the university you are considering attending. Your best option is a school with excellent academic programs that provide opportunities for contact with renowned scholars and world class scientists. You will need to be inspired by innovative programs of study presented by a committed, caring research faculty. A well-constructed work–life balance will add greatly to the value of your undergraduate education which should include mentorship opportunities and student life opportunities that are fun and compliment your academic science program.

3.2 THE VALUE OF DEPTH VS BREADTH IN YOUR UNDERGRADUATE CURRICULUM

As an undergraduate student, you are going to be faced with options for breadth and depth training. The former is provided as introductory and survey courses and is meant to expose you to several areas of study to provide you with a rounded education. The latter is designed to provide deep content expertise in a focused area thus providing the opportunity to carry out research projects and/or in-depth analysis of a topic leading to a project report/mini thesis. The in-depth route is an excellent preparation for graduate studies since it challenges you

> Specialist Programs Provide Excellent Platforms for Career Development

academically and shows potential supervisors that you have the capacity to explore complex problems and seek solutions. It is also flexible as it provides you with many problem-solving and analytical skills that are transferrable if you choose to move to other areas of study.

You may elect to strive for a combination, such as an in-depth specialist or honors program in one area and a major program in another to provide breadth. This may prepare you to carry out research as a graduate student and postdoctoral trainee at the interface of disciplines. Interdisciplinary research is now valued in biomedical and life sciences research to investigate and solve complex problems. Students are encouraged to work across disciplines and to be exposed to transdisciplinary and team approaches to problem solving. You will be expected to bring your in-depth knowledge to the table to tackle problems by learning from colleagues in other disciplines to look at a problem through many perspectives while also sharpening your own perspective.

The innovation of linking you as an undergraduate student with graduate students provides new transformative opportunities for your education. The link facilitates development of courses that are of value to both graduate and undergraduate students, such as a course on ethics and integrity in research. This approach allows for seamless integration of advanced senior undergraduate learning with graduate education and provides the much needed depth of scholarship to prepare undergraduates for advanced education. By having greater interaction with undergraduate students, graduate students have opportunities to mentor undergraduates. Undergraduate students are thus exposed to the innovation agenda of graduate education as well as to the best research faculty available to teach and mentor them.

| Achieve Seamless Transition from Undergraduate to Graduate Programs |

3.3 GUIDANCE IN SUCCESSFUL CAREER DEVELOPMENT

No one can advance along a career path alone and thus you should seek advice from professional career counselors, from individuals who are current practitioners of specific careers and most importantly from mentors. You will also need support from family, friends, and partners; however, they are too close to you so that they may be unable to remain neutral and may interject personal biases.

To provide career guidance, you should seek out people with intimate knowledge of biomedical and life science—associated careers and of the general area of career development. They will be able to provide the current best practice to the mechanics of career building. Often these are people you meet on occasion to obtain specific career information, such as on creating a CV, on seeking job

| Use Mentors Effectively and Wisely |

interviews, and on communication tips. You may hear them speak at a seminar or career symposium. This is important but not sufficient. Perhaps now as a novice undergraduate student it is a good time to discuss mentorship with you. Thinking ahead will require choosing and interacting with mentors.

3.4 THE VALUE OF A MENTOR

You need to find knowledgeable folks who are interested in you and in your succeeding in your academic pursuits. These are mentors who are usually teachers and professional life sciences researchers interested in undergraduate students. As you advance to graduate school and beyond, you may keep your mentors and add mentors who are closely aligned to careers that you are very interested in. Your mentors will advise you on pathways to follow, on opportunities to seek, and on how to prepare for these. Best practice is to seek more than one mentor since each will have specific qualities and expertise. Do not get into a situation where diametrically opposite views are expressed by different mentors as this will confuse you.

Mentors should consider themselves guides and sources of information, but they should leave the final choices to you. Their job is to open your eyes but not to live your life for you. Mentors should not be disappointed with your choices. They should feel proud in providing you with useful information and the guidance necessary for you to make your choices. Even at an early stage, seek out mentors who can help you with advice on how to deal with barriers that you may need to overcome as you move forward.

What do I look for in a mentee? I assess the interest the student has in me. This may be a strange consideration since they are the ones looking for advice. However, if the student has not checked me out and does not know who I am, what I do, and what my track record is in supervising and mentoring students, then the student may not be serious about developing this mentor–mentee relationship.

I have mentored many students both at the undergraduate and graduate level. I found that first and foremost I have to break down the barrier that exists between a professor and a student. We have to respect each other and interact as friends. I find it works best if the mentor is willing to learn from the mentee, especially about how students think and react to their environment. So each individual brings something to the table and benefits from the relationship. Once the introduction is over, I let the student know what areas I can help them with and in which areas they should look for additional mentors.

| The Mentor and the Mentee Learn from Each Other |

If they regard me as their primary mentor, they should keep me in the loop on major issues, even though these may be out of my area of expertise. I let the students know that we should meet regularly and that I am available anytime for urgent matters. I expect the mentee to attend meetings on time and to let me know if they are going to be late or must cancel. This is about respecting my time as a mentor. The best way to communicate is by face-to-face meetings at least a few times a year. E-mail can be used between meetings. For confidential matters, it is best to communicate face-to-face and not have random written records that may go astray.

As a mentor I am prepared to submit letters of reference and/or provide phone references. I do caution the student that I can only comment on what I know about them first hand. Thus if I never heard them make a presentation, I cannot provide an assessment on this area. Besides the obvious academic questions, recipients of referee comments frequently ask about the ability of the student to work in groups and to get along with peers and with faculty and staff. They are not interested in hiring someone who will be disruptive to their own group. They want to know if you are helpful to your peers and are willing to share in your work environment. They also want to know about the reliability of the student. Does the student arrive at meetings or seminars on time? Does the student let you know if they are going to be late or if they have to cancel their meeting? Other common referee questions are on motivation, creativity, innovation, and the willingness to engage in discussions and group projects.

As a mentor, I suggest opportunities for those whom I mentor, in a manner similar to the opportunities that were suggested to me when I was a trainee. This does not mean that you will get preferential treatment. It means that you are alerted to opportunities and it is up to you to follow through or not. For example, when my mentor was unavailable to teach his group of students, he asked me to substitute for him. I could have looked upon the request as an inconvenience. It was extra work and I had a full schedule. However, I recognized that this was an opportunity for me, so I taught and did well. This led to further teaching, and to working on curriculum development which later turned out to be one of my early duties as a faculty member, for which I was well prepared. In my case it was a true mentor–mentee collaboration that benefitted both parties.

3.5 HOW TO BEHAVE AS A MENTEE

As a mentee, put in the effort to select suitable mentors. You have to be serious about developing a mentor–mentee relationship. You should check out potential mentors by learning about the research work they carry out and their track record in training and mentoring students. You need to consider whether a potential mentor has the specific personal characteristics you seek in a mentor that would align with your own needs as a student and emerging scientist.

What you should consider before choosing your mentor(s) (not all issues are relevant to all mentee–mentor relationships):

- Do you prefer to be assigned a mentor or would you actively seek a mentor?
- Background training; where, type.
- Employment history, academic, and professional.
- Experience as a mentor, research supervisor, student advisory committee member.
- Understand the style of mentorship they use and assess whether this fits your expectations.
- Experience in your fields of interest with contacts in those communities.
- Views on work–life balance and on active career planning.
- Views on training in professional development.
- Understanding about gender issues, underrepresented and/or low-income communities. Having overcome these roadblocks a mentor may be in a better position to help you to navigate your path to success.
- Do you feel that you would seek emotional or psychological support from the individual?
- Do you feel you can establish a personal connection with this individual?

The mentee should expect that their mentors respect them, listen carefully to what they say, and provide a safe confidential environment for the mentorship interactions. The mentee should expect that their mentor is a nonjudgmental supporter of their career development and that their mentor promotes their successful training and career advancement.

> The Mentee Has Important Responsibilities

The mentee has responsibilities as well. The mentee should behave in a respectful manner and be mindful of the time and effort that the mentor is providing. The mentee should be honest with the mentor and keep them in the loop on matters related to their mentorship. The mentee should show appreciation and should be willing to assist the mentor as appropriate and in situations that provide benefits to both. The mentee should be available to provide evaluations of their mentors, such as for promotions and awards.

What I have found is that there are common themes that are much valued by undergraduate and graduate student mentees. This is apparent when they are asked to express critiques of their own supervisors and mentors. They value foremost when their academic supervisor is not only an excellent supervisor but also a nurturing mentor.

I find that students report in their evaluation letters of faculty teaching/mentorship that taking a nurturing interest in them beyond the immediate laboratory and research activities is highly valued. They praise faculty who are accessible to them for career development advice, who are interested in helping to advance their career aspirations. They value faculty who provide them with latitude to explore career options outside the wet bench environment and to take part in community activities such as student government, outreach programs to less advantaged communities, and advocacy programs for science. Some mentors I know show support of extracurricular activities by attending their student's artistic performances. I have found that students want more social contact with faculty. Students want to see faculty outside the classroom and laboratory. This helps to build peer relationships in addition to the standard hierarchal faculty—student relationship that occur in lectures and laboratories. Many students enjoy sports competitions. An annual faculty vs student sporting event is appreciated. In my own experience we had summer baseball. The department participated in a noncompetitive university league in which a departmental co-ed team was made up of faculty, administrative staff, and all levels of students.

Mentor—mentee relationships may last for the full course of your training and beyond. We have examples of mentors offering advice to the children of their mentees several years after the mentee has moved onto their own career. In most cases, however, the relationship may last until your training is completed and you secure your first job. When a mentor—mentee relationship turns into a friendship, as many of them do, you have harnessed the power of mentorship.

Besides these mentor—mentee relationships, I have received feedback from students on the value in creating a nurturing program or department that should be useful to academic leadership. The students are looking for the academic leadership of the department or program to create a nurturing environment where the culture includes caring for the well-being of all students. They are looking for a collegial community of scholars who will show an interest in what they think about their educational environment, and make them feel that they are part of the department. They are not just passing through for a few years but want to be considered part of the family—academically, intellectually, and socially.

> Students and Faculty Create Collegial Communities of Scholars

There is a group at the university that may provide an additional contribution to mentorship. These are the administrative staff who provide the infrastructure to run the courses, programs, visiting lecture series, student committee meetings, and student scholarship and award applications. It is common for students to go to administrative staff, i.e., the departmental undergraduate, graduate, or postdoctoral administrator for advice, both of a personal and professional nature. Once students leave the department for their next step, they often maintain these friendships with their favorite administrator.

Mentorship must be well done. It is becoming apparent in both academic and nonacademic institutions and businesses that evidence-based mentorship training programs are very useful to create and maintain a culture of mentorship within the organization. These educational programs need to have a well-defined curriculum and are usually first directed at the leadership of the organization who are in the best position to establish a culture of mentorship for students, trainees, faculty, and employees. Once the leadership is trained, these programs usually trickle down to those faculties who teach undergraduate, graduate, and postdoctoral students. These mentorship programs usually include development of evidence-based selection and evaluation processes to manage the mentorship activity in the department.

3.6 ACHIEVING VALUE IN YOUR UNDERGRADUATE MENTORED RESEARCH OPPORTUNITY

As an undergraduate student, you probably will be inspired by a lecture, a course, or a program which will help focus your research interest in life sciences and biomedical research. Speaking to professors, teaching assistants and peers will inform you about research opportunities that you could apply for. Many universities will have lists of undergraduate research opportunities on appropriate websites to make it easier for students to know what is available. Attending undergraduate student research presentations, departmental seminars, and reading the literature will open your eyes to interesting areas of research. Sometimes these experiences alert you very early on to an area of research that you would like to pursue. However, at this early stage the nature of the specific project you work on in the laboratory is less important than your learning the fundamentals of best practices in research in a nurturing laboratory environment.

> Undergraduate Research Laboratory Experience is Essential for Future Success

Research experience during your undergraduate program is critical in receiving future opportunities to be admitted to life sciences graduate programs. This experience may be obtained in credit courses that feature a research project or by mentored summer research opportunities (often not for credit) that have you immersed in a research laboratory doing hands-on work and functioning as a "junior" graduate student.

Having an awesome research experience will depend on both your own motivation and hard work, and the quality of the supervision you receive in the laboratory. Even for a short 12-week program, you will find it very useful to create an Undergraduate Diary which reflects competencies, milestones, and career development plans based on what is described below (Box 3.1). Prepare it with your mentor. This diary will guide you through these early defining

Box 3.1 Undergraduate Diary

Competencies, Milestones, and Career Plans

- Begin to write your Undergraduate Diary before you start your undergraduate program and update it as you progress in your course work, research experiences, and in your own ideas and goals.
- Discuss this document with your research supervisor and mentor. Update this undergraduate diary as you achieve each competency. Complete the full diary at the end of your program and research project. This will form the basis of future plans as you progress to graduate school or go out into industry.
- In comments, provide some details on each item including outcomes and future directions.
- Note that as you progress, career plans will be redesigned and rewritten at each major stage of your education, identifying new competencies to be achieved and milestones to be reached along the way. The career plan is a dynamic living document and is influenced by changes in both you and your environment.

Name:
Academic Status:
Date Diary Initiated:

A. Undergraduate Training

Supervisor(s):	Name
	Rank
	Department(s)

Mentor(s):	Name
	Rank
	Department(s)

Courses

1. Prerequisites
2. Undergraduate Program
3. Non-degree and non-university

B. Research
Complete a separate entry for each research project undertaken during your undergraduate studies.
   Dates of Research Project:
   Title of Project:

1. Why is your area of research important?
   Comment:
2. How is your project original, and what gap in knowledge are you try-ing to fill?
   Comment
3. What research skills will be critical to the success of your project?
   Comment:
4. Which meetings/conferences would be best suited for presentation of your project?
   Comment:
   a. Local
   b. Regional/National
   c. International
5. What journal(s) in your field would be best for publishing your work, and why?
   Comment:
6. How will this research project advance my career path?
   Comment

Research Qualifications and Certifications
Check the box if you have been exposed to and learned these skills and competencies during your research project

☐ **Code of Student Behavior**
   Comment:
☐ **Research Integrity Training**
   Comment:
☐ **Standard Operating Procedures in Biomedical/Life Sciences Laboratory**
   Comment:
☐ **Laboratory Health and Safety**
   Comment:
☐ **Animal Care Course/Procedures (as applicable)**
   Comment:
☐ **Human Research Ethics Training (as applicable)**
   Comment:

Research Skills and Competencies
☐ **Critical Reading of Literature**
   Comment:

☐ **Experimental Design**
Comment:
☐ **Technical Skills**
Comment:
☐ **Statistics, Computational Biology/Informatics (as applicable)**
Comment:
☐ **Analysis and Interpretation of Research Findings**
Comment:

Dissemination of Research Results
☐ **Informal Communication of Research**
    ☐ To Supervisor
    Comment:
    ☐ To Laboratory Group
    Comment:
    ☐ To Other Laboratories and Fellow Students in the Program
    Comment:
☐ **Poster Presentations**
    ☐ Local
    Comment:
    ☐ Elsewhere (Scientific Meeting)
    Comment:
☐ **Oral Presentations**
    ☐ Local
    Comment:
    ☐ Elsewhere (Scientific Meeting)
    Comment:
☐ **Writing Scientific Report or Abstract**
Comment:
☐ **Writing Manuscript for Publication**
Comment:
☐ **Prepare Elevator Pitch**

C. Career Planning and Development
☐ **Career Planning Lectures/Seminars (List)**
Comment:
☐ **Networking/Important Contacts**
Comment:
☐ **Exploring Graduate School Opportunities**
Comment:
☐ **Exploring Nonacademic Job Opportunities**
Comment:

Activities Outside the Research Laboratory:
- ☐ **Work–Life Integration**
  Comment:
- ☐ **Student Groups**
  Comment:
- ☐ **Outreach Programs**
  Comment:
- ☐ **Activities at University or elsewhere (sports/art/music/hobbies/other)**
  Comment:

Next Steps
Describe your next educational and career steps: Describe any changes in your career goals, e.g., courses, programs, and job experiences.

research years and provide a structure to record your adventure in undergraduate research.

3.7 MAKING THE MOST OF YOUR RESEARCH EXPERIENCE

You will experience and learn good laboratory practice including experimental design and analyses, critical evaluation, and communication and networking skills. You will also learn laboratory safety protocols and standard operating procedures. As you do your bench work, you need to learn how to properly document laboratory protocols you use and how to accurately record all of your laboratory experiments and activities. As you begin your research project, you will learn to design experiments, to use appropriate laboratory techniques, and to critically analyze and interpret data. Troubleshooting problems and actively formulating appropriate solutions is an important asset, and the undergraduate experience will start you down this road. As a trainee, you will learn how to search the scientific literature and learn how to critically evaluate scientific data and publications. You will communicate in a scholarly style, orally and in writing, through participation in seminars, written reports, journal articles, and poster presentations, including a final presentation of your research work. You will participate in journal clubs and/or laboratory meetings.

> Appreciate Advice on How to Get Better and Fine Tune Your Research Skills

An important pillar of career development is to learn to work as a team member in a collaborative research environment, and most but not all laboratories should provide you with this opportunity. As your project evolves, you will begin to build contacts with peers and professionals within your own research environment and beyond. Interdisciplinary and transdisciplinary research exposure will open your eyes to other perspectives that can shed light on your scientific problem.

During your time in the laboratory, take advantage of your supervisor, peers, especially senior undergraduates, graduate and postgraduate students, technicians, and those in neighboring laboratories to get feedback on your work and presentations. Being surrounded by smart, motivated peers and laboratory personnel helps to create high standards that inform your own work. At the end of your course, project, or summer experience, thank all those who helped you along the way. A well-written thank-you card is appreciated to acknowledge those who took the time and made the effort to support you in your research training.

Scientific societies and associations are creating opportunities for undergraduates to attend their scientific meetings and to present their research, usually as a poster presentation. In most cases as an undergraduate student, your research will involve collaboration from your laboratory. However, a reasonable portion should be done by you if you are going to present the work and write the abstract for the meeting. Attending these meetings in your own home town or elsewhere provides an exceptional opportunity to be part of a very important activity—the communication and discussion of scientific discovery with those who make the discoveries. Seek information and advice on how to prepare your presentation and how to present it at the meeting. Your supervisor and laboratory colleagues may help you rehearse your presentation and prompt you with likely questions you may be asked at the meeting. Students often ask me what to wear when they present. My response is neat, business casual attire in which you feel comfortable, especially if you need to stand by your poster. A colleague of mine tells her students to wear comfortable shoes when attending their poster.

The scientific societies usually set a very low registration fee for students and they may provide merit- and/or needs-based scholarships to support travel and board at the meeting. This is an excellent opportunity for you to gain confidence in presenting your work, to meet peers and scientists from other institutions, to hear and see excellent science, and to understand the culture and the community of science. Several of my students thoroughly enjoyed attending large scientific meetings and presenting their posters. They often meet researchers in the life sciences

> Undergraduates Benefit Attending Scientific Meetings

and biomedical field in which they are working and whose papers they had read. It was always a pleasure to see and hear the excitement in their voices when they described being interrogated at their poster by a "big name" in their field. This also gives them the chance to explore possible graduate positions. Senior faculty are always on the lookout for high-quality PhD candidates, so if you are interested in exploring programs outside your current institution, face-to-face contact with possible supervisors can occur at these meetings.

Even at this early undergraduate stage, you may be a student who will benefit from an international research experience which will broaden your horizons. This should be done carefully with advice from your university international experience office and with a thorough knowledge of the laboratory and institution you are planning to attend.

> International Research Experiences Should be Carefully Planned

You must pay attention to language requirements and to your ability to adapt to different scientific and personal cultures. As biomedical and life sciences become more global, a successful international experience can be very valuable as you plan your career.

Well Informed Decisions Result in a Quality Graduate Experience

CHAPTER 4

How to Select the Best Graduate Program for Your Needs

SUMMARY

You need to spend time and effort to select a graduate program that fits your needs. First through self-assessment and reflection you have to understand what your educational, scientific, and social needs are. Discuss with friends, family, and partners. Second, discuss your research goals with undergraduate mentors and professors. Then it is essential that you learn about the institution, program, and supervisor you are considering to do your graduate research with. Compare different graduate opportunities. The working relationship you have with your supervisor is critical to the success of your studies. Understand the style of training and the expectations a potential supervisor has. Does their style meet your own expectations and needs? Be sure to speak to many

Planning for a Career in Biomedical and Life Sciences. DOI: https://doi.org/10.1016/B978-0-12-814978-2.00004-1

students in your prospective programs to obtain information and opinions about the strengths and weaknesses of the program and of the supervisor you are considering. The quality of the students in the program will impact on the quality of your education and social experience. Moreover, ask more than just questions about the curriculum. Find out how the laboratory functions, how the supervisor interacts with students, and what resources the department/institution provides to enhance your educational experience. Are there opportunities for professional development? Try to obtain information regarding the faculty's level of contentment and the training program's cultural and social environment. Choose a research project from those offered to you by your own supervisor in either basic or translational science that is interesting to you and that explores an important gap in knowledge that if studied will provide exciting new findings that are publishable in top tier journals. When finally selecting a program, supervisor, and research question, understand the competencies that you need to achieve and the milestones you need to meet so that you can develop a comprehensive graduate career development plan.

You need to be well informed when selecting a graduate program, and this takes time and effort on your part. There are three levels you need to investigate: the institution, the program/department, and the research supervisor. You should begin your search no later than at the very beginning of fourth year undergraduate. In some instances, scholarship applications are due to be submitted in the early part of the fourth year. Make sure you are aware of the deadlines.

You may begin with a general search using the Internet to browse through local and distant opportunities. This overview gives you a sense of what programs are offering. Once you pare down your list, you need to do an in-depth look at several programs to be able to eventually select the best ones for you. If you are lucky, you already have identified your scientific passion. Have fun exploring it. You may even have identified a supervisor you wish to work with in your chosen area of research. However, like most undergraduate students, you may need to investigate several types of research before you settle on ones you wish to pursue. Your search should determine which programs offer you the right fit. You decide what you want out of the program and determine if you suit the program and the program suits you. A best fit requires that four components fit well: the student, the supervisor, the research environment, and the career plan (Fig. 4.1).

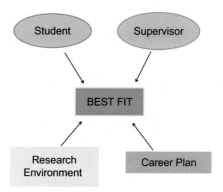

Figure 4.1 Choosing the right program and supervisor.

It is critical that you are well aware of the processes and deadlines that are in place for each program you apply to. They will vary as will documents you need to submit. Leave

| Be Aware of Application Processes and Deadlines |

yourself sufficient time to apply, especially to obtain letters of reference, transcripts, and as well as applications for internal and external scholarships as required.

4.1 ASSESSMENT OF THE QUALITY OF THE PROGRAM

| Identify High Quality Programs |

Assessment of academic quality is important but not simple. Often the students use the reputation of the institution as the indicator of quality. However, you need to dig deeper. The quality of the institution as a whole can be assessed by data on outcomes and impact of graduates. This is important and should be available to potential students. There are university ranking systems which provide rankings based on institutionally supplied data or data based on third-party sources. Each has its own problems in tackling this complex ranking issue. You have to be careful of aggregate ranking since it may not reflect the quality of the specific program you are interested in and may simply reflect the standing of the whole university or institution. Quality is often measured by the amount of research funding a department/program attracts and the quality of the publications of its members.

The quality of programs is enriched by having a smart, motivated, and diverse student body. This provides for friendly competition and sets high standards. Many students tell me that they learned much from their peers during their graduate training. Diversity of interests and of previous experiences promotes cross-fertilization of ideas by students from different undergraduate backgrounds as they come together as a community of graduate students. This opportunity to be exposed to and carry out research in an environment that values diversity is an important feature in your training.

> Student Advisory Committees Are Essential

4.2 IMPORTANT INFORMATION TO GATHER ON PROGRAMS

- Have you obtained a clear description of the full program offered to you?
- Have core competencies for your program been identified and clearly communicated to you?
- Are courses relevant to your research interests available to you?
- Are there opportunities for students to interact and work together?
- Is there a critical mass of highly qualified trainees in the program and in the institution as a whole?
- Does the program provide opportunities for formal presentations of your research during your training?
- Is there a strong policy with respect to student advisory committees and student mentoring? This is important since members of the committee help keep projects on track, provide expert advice on troubleshooting, may provide training with new techniques, and are an excellent source of reference letters.
- Does the program and/or institution have well-defined policies on training and graduate education, e.g., ethical conduct in research, intellectual property guidelines, publication policy, invention policy, safety policy, code of behavior on academic matters, graduate supervision policy and guidelines, effective mentorship program, and career counseling?
- Does the institution/department offer you co-curriculum programs/ graduate professional skills programs which augment the education you receive in your biomedical discipline?
- Are there faculty seminar series and visiting lectureships organized for your benefit?

- Does the department have a culture of innovation and entrepreneurial commercialization?
- Does the department/institution have opportunities to provide real-work experience for you including paid work term placements?
- What is the expected time to completion for graduate students in your program?
- Does the culture of the institution/department foster appropriate life–work balance for you to promote personal, professional, and emotional development?
- Are there successful departmental and institutional student groups and clubs available to you?
- Even as a student, are there opportunities for you to become part of the fundamental fabric of the department/institution?

4.3 PAYING ATTENTION TO PERSONAL ISSUES

Some of this information should be available on appropriate websites; however, the information should be verified and expanded in discussion with potential supervisors and program directors. Personal issues include salary, benefits, sick time, and health insurance. You should be very clear on student stipends including amounts, taxes, number of years covered, and availability of holiday time, meeting time, and book, computer/laptop, and travel allowances. You should know if you have to apply for competitive internal and/or external student funding. The institution should have programs that provide you with a safe and healthy work environment. If you live on campus, the buildings and walkways should be safe 24/7. In science, since you may work into the night, availability of food services after hours is useful.

If you will be residing off campus, living in an attractive safe neighborhood makes life pleasant for you and your family. Explore housing issues and possible institutional housing. Consider how much time you may be commuting. Institutions should have dedicated individuals to help with information on available services and relocation issues.

> Lifestyle Is Critical

> Consider Partner and Family Needs as You Plan Your Training

Involve your family in the decision-making. The quality of life in the city you choose to train in is an important issue to explore carefully. It is very important to make the training journey fun, so keep this in mind when making your choices.

4.4 CONSIDERATIONS OF FAMILY ISSUES

- Does the location allow you to have the quality of life you desire?
- What resources does the department or the institution have that promote the care and well-being of you and your family?
- If you have a spouse (partner) and a family, are their needs well met? If the family is not happy, you as a trainee will have an added burden. A presence of a nurturing community for the family is important, even if you stay in a location for only a few years.
- Do you need day care or schools?
- What educational programs are available for partners?
- What jobs are available for partners?

If you need to train for two careers, make sure the institution is able and willing to provide for the academic needs of the couple. Institutions are becoming much more aware of this need for dual careers and should be willing and able to discuss this with you and make appropriate accommodations.

4.5 WHAT TO BE AWARE OF IN CHOOSING INTERNATIONAL STUDIES

Some of you may wish to do a graduate degree at an international location. You may wish to continue in an area that you have been working in or you may wish to strike out in a new direction. In fact, certain projects are best done at international locations because of the nature of the work. You may be attracted to the institution because of its outstanding reputation or you may wish to work with a specific scientist whose work you admire. Be well informed. You must research your choices very carefully to ensure that you understand the educational characteristics of the institution that you plan to attend and the features it offers that will allow you to fit in well. You must be aware of the nature of the training and of the relationship that is expected between you and your supervisor and between you and your laboratory colleagues. These relationships are often related to the cultural norms that govern society and scientific research at your international location. There will be differences, often striking, between your current institution and department and the potential international site. While at your undergraduate university, discuss your options with a university office dedicated to international experiences and seek out students and faculty who can give you firsthand information and advice on institutions that you are considering. A visit to an international location is an excellent idea but it is not always possible. You meet/visit your supervisor, your fellow students, and see the environment in both department and institution. The consideration of studying in another geographic and cultural environment is very appealing; however, your main concern is that you live and work in a safe environment and receive a high-quality education that will indeed further your career aspirations.

4.6 HOW TO SELECT YOUR SUPERVISOR

Be well informed—spend the time necessary to obtain the information you need. Meet and get to know your potential supervisor, her trainees, and laboratory staff as best you can. Especially if you are coming from elsewhere, it is very valuable to visit your potential supervisor, and to meet laboratory trainees and staff as well. Make sure to see and explore the laboratory facility and the institution as a whole.

When obtaining information from your potential peers, contact as many trainees as possible to get a consensus opinion. You will find some trainees who are satisfied with everything and some who can see no good in anything in the program. What you need is a balanced view, and to get this you need to ask probing questions and try to get specific answers, not general impressions. This information you will collect is subjective but is very useful if you speak to enough people. Try to get a sense of the level of contentment within the student population as well as the faculty. Happy faculty tend to be much more inclined to create a healthy and exciting environment for training and supervision.

Choosing the right supervisor requires work on your part to ask the right questions. This one-on-one relationship with your supervisor is of paramount importance to the success of your graduate training. Personalities are

| Choosing the Best Supervisor and Laboratory for You is a Critical Decision |

important, so learn about your potential supervisor's personality and make sure it will mesh with yours. Both the working and personal relationship you have with your supervisor are very important. Where you may have co-supervisors, it is important that the three of you are on the same page. You should not function as a referee between two co-supervisors but instead, be part of a team that has all members pulling in the same direction.

In many cases, supervisors are not assigned to you by the program. Potential students are accepted into the program on condition that they find a supervisor. Thus potential trainees choose from a list of faculty who have positions available in that given year. Alternatively you may apply to a program specifically to work with a given supervisor. You may have worked under the supervisor as an undergraduate and/or you may be attracted by the reputation of the supervisor or the area of study. When choosing from a list of research supervisors, visit the laboratory and talk to the current trainees. Review the supervisor's CV, especially publications and grants. The quality and impact of the publications and the size and number of grants are most important. Try to find out the scientific reputation of potential supervisors.

> The Working Relationship With Your Supervisor Is Important

A very useful recruitment model that many departments offer is that once you are accepted to the program, the program provides rotations to make it easier for you to choose a laboratory to train in. When you begin your training, these programs provide several short electives/rotations in a few laboratories that are of interest to you. In most cases, you will end up choosing one of these rotation laboratories to do your research thesis in, since you have had a firsthand opportunity to experience the laboratory and work with the supervisor.

The philosophy and the curriculum of the training program should support and value high-quality research opportunities in the laboratory you choose to work in. Your supervisor should maintain a culture that is free from harassment and discrimination. It should be a nurturing environment. This should be supported by specific policies that are enforced. Current and former student experiences in these areas provide you with very useful information.

4.7 A THOROUGH LIST OF QUESTIONS THAT REQUIRE ANSWERS FROM YOUR POTENTIAL SUPERVISOR AND/OR STUDENTS IN THE LABORATORY

- How does your potential supervisor run the laboratory and the research program?
- Is the laboratory well-funded?
- Is there sufficient space and equipment?
- How much contact time does your supervisor provide you for research supervision?
- How often will formal meetings be held with your supervisor?
- Does the supervisor provide constructive feedback in a timely manner?
- How often will you meet with your student advisory committee and are these committees effective?
- Is there adequate assessment of your progress in course work and research?
- Do students finish their program in a timely fashion (often referred to as "time to completion")?
- Are journal clubs part of the laboratory activity?
- Are there visiting scientists presenting seminars and interacting with students?
- Does the supervisor have international colleagues and collaborators?
- Does the supervisor actively mentor students in career development especially with personal development plans?
- Do students publish first-authored high-quality work?
- How do current students in the laboratory assess the strength and weaknesses of their supervisor?

It is indeed important to have an open discussion with a potential supervisor to get your questions answered and receive the information you need to make an informed choice. If you are unable to have this discussion, this may not be the laboratory for you to train in.

4.8 STUDENT VIEWS OF GRADUATE SUPERVISORS

A five-star research supervisor according to many students is one who sits down often to discuss your research project, who provides access to technical expertise, and who guides you but does not necessarily micromanage you through your research project. Students report that they like to try new approaches or ideas out in the laboratory and enjoy this latitude. They want to be supported in both their successes and their failures at the bench. Some students like some active participation of their supervisor in the wet laboratory. They like to work side by side with their supervisor. In reality, this will happen much more often with a young faculty member, and less so with a more senior investigator since the latter will have more nonlaboratory duties and activities to attend to in her department, institution, and discipline. Students also appreciate when their supervisor is available to them outside formal meetings, so that when a research issue comes up, they can deal with it quickly. Supervisors who are easily accessible are lauded for this characteristic. Students appreciate quick feedback on reports and on applications that they are preparing, for example, for studentships, scholarships, and awards. Students also appreciate a supervisor who actively facilitates their contact with other investigators and their laboratory groups, so that they can learn new techniques that they need for their research project. Students also appreciate the time faculty spend on student advisory committees and on volunteering to judge poster and oral research presentations.

> Research Supervisors Have Different Styles of Training and Expectations

Many students, in reference letters written about their own supervisor, value being asked to help review a manuscript or a grant application that their supervisor has received. Students regard this activity in a positive way in helping to sharpen their critical skills and teaching them how to write their own manuscripts and research grants. They view this as a confidence building activity as well since their experienced supervisor trusts them to carry out this important task and is eager to hear their own critical opinion on science. This should not be viewed by students as dumping more work on their plate. The value of course is in the discussions that follow with the supervisor where the students obtain feedback on their critical views.

4.9 HOW TO CHOOSE YOUR RESEARCH PROJECTS

Once you have identified your supervisor, you will discuss different projects with your supervisor and after considering them, you will pursue one. To help make your decision you should read the relevant literature pertaining to the research project so that you are making an informed choice. One of our students noted that he chose a project on inflammation because as an undergraduate, he realized that inflammation signal pathways were very important in several disease states. Thus he realized this topic was important and presented numerous opportunities for innovative studies. Another chose to work on Alzheimer disease because he watched one of his close relatives live with this disease, and this sparked his interest and his desire to contribute to understanding the condition and developing possible therapies. Although you will have choices as to

Work on an Important Gap in Knowledge

which knowledge gaps you wish to pursue, your project should be one that your supervisor is very interested in and that fits well with the overall program of the laboratory. The project should also interest you and be challenging enough so that there is a high probability of success in completing innovative work that is publishable in a high-impact journal. The project should result in an excellent life sciences/biomedical written thesis. You will be required to defend the research at a thesis defense with an oral presentation and an in-depth defense of your work in front of a committee of knowledgeable faculty, both internal and external to your institution.

The scientist's challenge is to design clever experiments to reveal the cell's secrets. Remember that research is unpredictable. You spend a considerable amount of time reading and thinking about a biological question before you decide on an approach to test a hypothesis that will provide you with new knowledge. What can be more daunting and, at the same time, more fun than identifying a biological question that you find exciting? You have the opportunity to design and plan experiments that will try to explain the biology that so fascinates you. You get to carry out the investigation. You decide what techniques you need to use and learn how to use them correctly and safely. Then you carry out the experiments, troubleshooting any technical issues that get in your way. To make sure you have it right, you repeat the experiments several times until you are certain all is well. This may be tedious but essential for research integrity. You analyze the data carefully using the best qualitative and quantitative methods. Once you are confident of the validity of the data, you interpret your findings. Is it new? Can you explain what you have found based on what is known from other experiments published in the literature? Most often the results of experiments raise new questions prompting you to explore your biological problem at a deeper and deeper level.

Looking at the same old problem in a fresh way—we call this thinking outside the box—is an exciting way to tackle a scientific problem. It is not uncommon to gain some sudden insight into a problem that you are investigating in the laboratory while carrying out some unrelated tasks outside the laboratory at home or on vacation. As long as your problem is imbedded in your mind, insights may indeed come from the strangest places. There are many examples of this in science. Insight is often the product of a prepared mind.

4.10 TRANSLATING DISCOVERY RESEARCH

You now want to take your basic science discoveries and translate them into products or treatments that have medical and societal benefits for individuals and communities. You may focus on a disease or on a communal or global scientific problem such as global nutrition or child and women's health. The general path is from initial basic discovery to the development of a diagnostic, prevention, or treatment tool which is tested successfully in clinical trials and then is utilized in regular clinical practice. This is the "bench to bedside" pathway of translational research.

Although graduate research does not span a long period of time and is being carried out by relative newcomers to the field, some trainees are able to initiate the bench to bedside pathway by discovering new knowledge that has a reasonable potential to produce a new treatment or a new drug/device that impacts health care. In some projects it is serendipity that results in an innovative finding, and in others the research plan is designed from the onset to discover new knowledge that has potential for clinical benefit. In the latter case the student and supervisor have a well-developed research question and the resources and technology at hand to carry the entrepreneurial project forward. They also understand the societal need for their product. Thus, should the research be successful, there is a good chance of establishing a commercialization pathway and attracting investment to support moving forward with early product development.

Depending on the length of time the discovery research takes, there may not be time to carry out even some initial steps in product development during the PhD studies and thesis work. Thus this work will follow after the degree is granted. At this point, the student has to make a choice after she gets her degree. Does she want to continue developing the finding along a translational paradigm, or does she want to hand it off at this point and move on with her own life sciences training? She may remain minimally involved. Issues around intellectual property have to be carefully considered with those involved at the university and/or institution. Alternatively, she may wish to continue to develop her finding. This will likely require new experiments and acquiring new skill sets and mentors familiar with product development and commercialization. This is a long process and usually involves several years of work. Universities and research institutes have developed infrastructures such as incubator facilities to assist students in the early stages of these endeavors, creating effective innovation ecosystems to advance the translation and commercialization agenda.

Hard Work, Self-Reflection, Resilience and New Knowledge Go Hand in Hand in Career Development

CHAPTER 5

Life in the Research Laboratory

SUMMARY

The life sciences/biomedical research laboratory is an ecosystem into which you need to fit comfortably. To do this, observe carefully and learn the culture and the dynamics of your laboratory group. You will have your input into the culture but do not expect the culture to change to fit your own needs. Become a team player, interact with peers, technicians, faculty, and staff and be ready for both scientific and social interactions. Manage your time well, share ideas and knowledge, be helpful, and do your share of general laboratory upkeep. Learn how to run experiments and keep comprehensive accurate records. Develop communication skills to prepare for meetings with your supervisor and your student advisory committee. Read the literature and learn to be critical in a positive way. Failure and rejection is a frequent occurrence so learn to be resilient. Learn and utilize coping skills and do not hesitate to consult your mentors and your supervisor for assistance at stressful

Planning for a Career in Biomedical and Life Sciences. DOI: https://doi.org/10.1016/B978-0-12-814978-2.00005-3

moments. Be prepared to learn from your failures and rejections which helps you bounce back even stronger than you were. As you progress forward in your research work, you will gain more confidence and begin to see satisfying results from your hard labor. Life science research is hard work and is most often not predictable, so adapt to this and enjoy your journey of discovery. Keep your graduate career development plan up to date so that you can monitor your progress and make alterations as you and your environment inevitably change over time. The career plan will also help you focus on professional skills that enhance your scientific laboratory training.

5.1 BUILDING YOUR CONFIDENCE

Begin by preparing your Graduate Career Development plan, in consultation with your supervisor and mentors (Box 5.1). You are entering a new environment, or even if it is your former undergraduate department, you will be looking at it with a new pair of eyes, those of a graduate student. Initially, graduate training can be an overwhelming experience. You face several challenges which may be stressful. You need to find your way around the institution. You have to define/stake out your space in your new laboratory and office. First interactions with your lab mates may be difficult. You begin to identify which peers can help you and mentor you in these early days to help build your confidence. Do not be shy to ask them questions. You begin to learn protocols and techniques and how the laboratory runs. You will make mistakes and have to repeat experiments. Sometimes you may inadvertently alter the steps in the protocol or you forget to add a reagent. You may incubate for too short a time or too long a time. Eventually, the mistakes become much less frequent. As a graduate student, you will recognize that your skills, maturity, and confidence will improve steadily over time.

Very early on, you need to develop sound time management skills and learn to multitask efficiently and effectively. Many students find it very useful to prepare a detailed schedule for the upcoming week for themselves. This helps guide and focus their work and provides very short-term milestones. This too will build your confidence by providing you with solid work approaches and very good time management.

Manage Your Time Well

Box 5.1 Graduate Career Development Plan

Plans, Competencies, and Milestones

- Career development plans should be designed and rewritten at each major stage of your education, identifying competencies to be achieved and milestones to be reached along the way.
- Begin your individual career development plan before you start your graduate program and your research project. These go hand-in-hand as you chart the present and the future. Discuss the plan with your research supervisor. The plan is a dynamic living document.
- Update this graduate plan as you achieve each competency and achieve a milestone. Complete the full plan at the end of your project. This will form the basis of future plans.
- In comments, provide some details on each item including outcomes and future directions.

Graduate Training

Name:
    Academic Status:
    Date Plan Initiated:

Supervisor(s):   Name
                 Rank
                 Department(s)
Mentor(s):   Name
                 Rank
                 Department(s)

Student Advisory Committee Members (List with brief comment on expertise):

Courses

1. Prerequisites
2. Graduate Program
3. Graduate Professional Development (non-degree or non-university)

Teaching/Mentoring Experience

☐ Teaching Assistant
   Comment:
☐ Tutor
   Comment:
☐ Mentoring Students
   Comment:
☐ Other
   Comment:

Research Project
Title of Project

1. Why is your area of research important?
   Comment:
2. How is your project original, and what gap in knowledge are you try-ing to fill?
   Comment:
3. What research skills will be critical to the success of this project?
   Comment:
4. Which meetings/ conferences would be best suited for presentation of your project?
   Comment:
   a. Local
   b. Regional/National
   c. International
5. What journal(s) in your field would be best for publishing your work, and why?
   Comment:

Research Qualifications and Certifications
Check the box when you learned these skills and competencies

- ☐ **Code of Student Behavior**
  Comment:
- ☐ **Research Integrity Training**
  Comment:
- ☐ **Standard Operating Procedures in Biomedical/Life Sciences Laboratory**
  Comment:
- ☐ **Laboratory Health and Safety**
  Comment:
- ☐ **Animal Care Course/Procedures (as applicable)**
  Comment:
- ☐ **Human Research Ethics Training (as applicable)**
  Comment:

Research Skills and Competencies
- ☐ **Critical Reading of Literature**
  Comment:
- ☐ **Experimental Design**
  Comment:
- ☐ **Technical Skills**
  Comment:
- ☐ **Analysis and Interpretation of Research Findings**
  Comment:

☐ **Computational Biology/Informatics**
Comment:

Dissemination of Research Results
☐ **Informal Communication of Research**
  ☐ To Supervisor
  Comment:
  ☐ To Laboratory Group
  Comment:
  ☐ To Other Laboratories and Fellow Students in the Program
  Comment:
☐ **Poster Presentations**
  ☐ Local/Away (e.g., Scientific Meeting)
  Comment:
☐ **Oral Presentations**
  ☐ Local/Away (e.g., Scientific Meeting)
  Comment:
☐ **Writing Scientific Report or Abstract**
Comment:
☐ **Writing Manuscript for Publication**
Comment:
☐ **Project Abstract (250 words) for each presentation/poster**
☐ **Abstract of Final Thesis**
☐ **Elevator Pitch (prepare a 60-second pitch)**

Milestones (Include Expected Date and When Achieved)
☐ **Committee Meetings (every eight months)**
Comment:
☐ **Comprehensive Exam (as applicable)**
Comment:
☐ **Seminar Presentations**
Comment:
☐ **Completion of Courses**
Comment:
☐ **Submission of Manuscript(s)**
Comment:
☐ **Publication of Manuscript(s)**
Comment:
☐ **Permission to Write up Thesis**
Comment:
☐ **Thesis Defense**
Comment:

Activities Outside the Laboratory
☐ **Student Groups**
Comment:
☐ **Outreach Programs**
Comment:
☐ **Activities at University or Elsewhere**
　☐ Sports
　Comment:
　☐ Music/Art
　Comment:
　☐ Hobbies
　Comment:
　☐ Other
　Comment:

Preparing for Next Steps While in Graduate Program
☐ **Laboratory Management Skills**
Comment:
☐ **Leadership Skills**
Comment:
☐ **Career Planning Lectures/Seminars (List Those Attended); Graduate Professional Development**
Comment:
☐ **Learning about Careers in Academic, Private, Public, and Non-Profit Sectors**
Comment:
☐ **Short Internship to Sample Careers**
Comment:
☐ **Networking/Important Contacts**
Comment:

Next Steps
☐ **Postdoctoral Research Training**
Comment:
☐ **Job Searches/Applications/Resume**
Comment:

5.2 TIPS ON DEVELOPING PEOPLE SKILLS

Learning to work with colleagues is essential in life sciences and biomedical research since research requires assistance from others. You are working in a community of scientists. Your community is first and foremost your own laboratory. This may be small with a few people or it may be large with several students, postdoctoral students, research associates, technicians, and staff. You have to be able to function efficiently and effectively within the laboratory setting. You may be sharing laboratory bench space, equipment, imaging stations, etc., and you need to learn how to be firm and accommodating at the same time. Do not book time on a piece of equipment for several days at a time which prevents colleagues and peers from doing their work. Discuss with users of the equipment how best to satisfy everyone's needs in the laboratory. If you see that you will not be using equipment that you booked, remove your name immediately from the time sheet and let colleagues know so that they may take advantage of this free time. If you are using common equipment or equipment in a colleague's laboratory, do not overstay your welcome and make sure you know how to use the equipment so that you do not inadvertently take it out of service. Clean up after you use the equipment and replace any supplies so that the next person does not have to scramble to get supplies just as they are ready to use the equipment. Report any malfunctions immediately so that they may be fixed and others are not disadvantaged. To use some heavily used equipment, you may need to stay after hours; however, these early or late time slots should be distributed among the group of users.

On the personal side, say "good morning" or "have a good evening/weekend." Smile and do not be grumpy. Say please and thank you, especially when folks do you a favor.

> Be a Collegial Lab Mate

Sometimes a colleague needs a helping hand in a complex experiment, so be ready and willing to lend a hand. The laboratory environment is a close contact environment so that being courteous and considerate is important in making life in the science laboratory pleasant and fun for all.

5.3 THE IMPORTANCE OF RECORD KEEPING

As you work in the laboratory, you must be aware of and document that you are carrying out the best scientific procedures and are following the highest ethical research standards. You must learn to keep a laboratory book which chronicles your daily activities in the laboratory. These books are reviewed by your supervisor and available for audit by others outside the laboratory. Some laboratories use a homegrown or commercial electronic research laboratory notebook.

Experiments should be well described, including animal experiments. You must have animal care approval by the institution's animal care committee and have taken animal care training offered by the institution. You cannot begin experiments before training and approvals are completed. Data should be meticulously kept. Preservation of data is at the core of the highest standards of ethical conduct in research. All entries must include dates. The page numbers of the laboratory books must be inscribed consecutively. The book should be kept in a safe place in the laboratory, so entries can be made in real time and the book does not get lost or misplaced in transit out of the laboratory. Original data and images and all data analysis must be kept well organized so that they are readily available for review or audit purposes. Every image or graph you keep for your records should be of publication quality. All your original data should be encrypted so that it is secure and, if lost, remains secure. Back up all your data. If you are using any data or information or studies that involve people, be very familiar with your institution's rules and guidelines for handling human research information, including requirements for human research ethics board approvals. Research involving humans must be approved before any experimentation may commence and the protocols, once approved, must be followed meticulously as per the conditions of the approval. Any changes in protocol require review by the board.

Keep Comprehensive Accurate Lab Books

5.4 PREPARING FOR SUPERVISOR MEETINGS

Initially you may find that meeting with your supervisor to discuss your work is intimidating. It is helpful to send an e-mail with your data to your supervisor ahead of time. She will have time to think about your work before you meet. It is best to be well prepared. Consider what you want to convey and what help you need to ask for. Be open and address issues in a clear comprehensive way showing all the data, the good and the not so good. Do not use the term "you are not going to like the data." What you are saying is that the data does not fit the hypothesis and your supervisor is going to be unhappy. However your supervisor should accept this, as long as your experiments are well designed, carried out, analyzed, and interpreted. You should take control of your

Be Well Prepared for Meetings with your Supervisor

project—it is your project. Be confident. No one should know as much as you do about your own project but remember that everyone needs input and advice both initially and as your work evolves.

Once your research begins, you need to discuss authorship and the institution's policies on intellectual property with your supervisor. You should understand what intellectual input and work is required to claim first authorship, which in life sciences means you are the senior author. Your supervisor then becomes the senior responsible author and usually the corresponding author. Problems are more likely to arise when more than one graduate student and more than one principal investigator are involved in the project. Then a plan for authorship should be drawn up in writing to avoid arguments and misunderstandings that might come up later. The original plan may change as the research progresses and experiments are added or deleted. This should be done to everyone's satisfaction. Sometimes you may need a neutral opinion, such as that of a graduate coordinator to help resolve authorship issues.

5.5 USING YOUR STUDENT ADVISORY COMMITTEE TO YOUR BEST ADVANTAGE

In most graduate programs a student advisory committee is a requirement of the program, and if it is not, then it should be. There are departmental/institutional guidelines to inform the student, supervisor, and committee members on the role of the committee, how to conduct the meetings, and what to expect from them. The membership of the committee should be established as soon as possible, within six months of starting the program. The frequency of the meetings should be about every eight months with the first occurring to meet the student and hear a presentation and report on the background, the research plans, and a few preliminary experiments.

> Use Your Student Advisory Committee Well

The committee usually includes the supervisor and two or three faculty members. The committee members should be chosen by you in consultation with your supervisor, and they should be free of conflict. The department may require that one member be from another department. The members should have the scientific expertise to provide you with advice and to assess the progress of your work. This requires that the committee evaluate your work but the meeting is not an evaluation process. The evaluation is to assess progress and determine if you are achieving research competencies. Some students have told me that they regard a committee meeting as the "day of judgment." It should not be so. The atmosphere should be collegial, warm, and friendly. Usually a typical meeting will begin with a presentation by you, the student, with emphasis on experimental design, execution of experiments, data analysis, and conclusions. You should prepare a full report for distribution to your supervisor and committee members seven to ten days before the meeting. The report should be well done, so take the time to compose drafts and obtain feedback from your peers and your supervisor on the makeup of the report. A committee meeting is a time and place to put your best foot forward in a protected environment. Your presentation is followed by a general roundtable discussion which should focus on the presentation and report. Your supervisor should allow you to engage in the full discussion. Where it is necessary and appropriate, your supervisor should contribute. On occasion, there is considerable cross-talk between committee members and the supervisor. This is not helpful for you. You need to ask questions of your committee members and discuss conceptual and technical issues that are on your mind. It is important as well to present and discuss experiments that did not work. To your surprise, you may get useful feedback on the failures as well. There is usually a report of the meeting, often a template created by the department/program to be filled out and signed by all parties. Helpful comments on the research, suggestions on the future direction of the work, and the goals and outcomes to be achieved by the next meeting should be clearly described in the report and agreed upon by you, your supervisor, and committee members. The committee members may often be willing to have you come to their laboratory to refine and/or learn new techniques that will be helpful for your research. Although the overall tone of the student advisory committee meeting should be collegial and supportive of your efforts, committee members are most effective when they provide you with an honest critique of your research work. The emphasis should be to guide you in your work, and to do so you must provide the members with all your work and have raw data available, especially if there are questions on the analysis of the data. If your progress is lagging this should be made clear to you and suggestions on how to improve progress must be included in the report. Time to completion of your thesis work is

> Your Advisory Committee Meeting is a Protected Environment

> Learn from Critical Analysis of Your Work

important and the committee should provide direction to you on how to advance your project at an appropriate pace.

Committee members should be available to you outside of the meeting format for advice between meetings. Some students find a one-on-one meeting a very useful addition to the process. A committee member may also be able to mentor you as well, although many students prefer the two tasks to be separated. As your project progresses, you and your supervisor may wish to add another member to the committee, usually to provide needed scientific expertise. On occasion you may find that a member is no longer useful as your project moves forward. You should discuss this with your supervisor and perhaps a change is required. Your committee members will get to know you, so they may be fine sources of letters of reference for awards/scholarship applications, postdoctoral applications, and job applications.

It is the committee members, in consultation with your supervisor, who determine what constitutes an appropriate thesis for you. This decision-making process occurs when your research work is complete and ready to write up as a thesis. You are then granted permission to write up your thesis and once done, defend your work at your thesis defense. The format of the thesis defense will vary from department to department and institution to institution. Most universities require an external (to the university) examiner and a thesis committee made up of members from the department and from cognate departments.

5.6 KNOW THE LITERATURE

Read the literature extensively, critically, and in a timely fashion. Keep up-to-date and learn to search the literature accurately. Most graduate programs offer seminars on how to effectively search the literature. You should not let articles pile up because it is very difficult to catch up. This is very important and is essential to carry out and interpret your own research work and to broaden your general biomedical and life sciences knowledge base. Stay current and be ready to discuss the latest breakthroughs in your own field and in science in general. You should be providing new interesting articles to your supervisor and to your peers. Spend time to maintain your literature references well organized and easily accessible.

> Be Current with Your Reading of the Research Literature

5.7 ACQUIRING COMMUNICATION SKILLS

Seize every opportunity to improve your ability to communicate effectively. You should be learning how to write scientific abstracts and articles and to present short and standard-length scientific talks. Be sure to obtain feedback on all your efforts. Communication can always be improved upon, so be open to constructive criticism. Some institutions provide face-to-face and/or online modules to train students in communication techniques. While in graduate school, pay attention to these "soft skills" and make sure that you communicate well, both orally and in writing, that you learn to network, and that you learn how to communicate with peers and colleagues at those scientific meetings that you attend. The latter is very important and helps you to meet scientists in your field and to begin to build your scientific reputation.

An important term that you will hear is the "elevator pitch." This refers to a scenario where you are riding an elevator with someone and you have about 30 seconds to answer the question she poses to you—"What exactly is it that you do?" The

Prepare an Effective Elevator Pitch

question is meant to illicit an honest comprehensible response to someone who may be interested in what you have to say. Thus you have to be able to provide key information in a succinct manner that is clear and focuses on highlights rather than details. One approach is to create a template for yourself that begins with the reason you are doing this type of project, and then includes the hypothesis you are testing, the

Prepare Business Cards for Yourself

methods you use, the new knowledge that you have generated or hope to generate, and the importance of the discovery to the listener and to the community as a whole. You end by offering to provide more information at a later date perhaps by handing them your business card. Your hope is that they recognize you as a confident individual, that they are interested in what you said, and that they can see the importance of the research. The listener asks herself "what does this mean to me? How does your work relate to my interests?" If you are very successful, they will ask for more information, perhaps by requesting your business card if you have not yet given it to them, so that they can further communicate with you. It is very hard to come up with an elevator pitch on the spot. You need to prepare the pitch, refine it, and have it well-rehearsed so that you can deliver it in the

30 second time slot when the opportunity arises. As you become more experienced, you may spontaneously tailor a sentence that is specifically relevant to the listener, if you know something about this person. This pitch is important when you speak to potential postdoctoral supervisors, academic and nonacademic recruiters, potential collaborators, network buddies, and science funders, especially those from non-government agencies, industry, and philanthropies. The pitch is to get your foot in the door. If the listener is interested, you will have the opportunity to provide much more detail at a later date. The elevator pitch is analogous to "speed dating" in the social scene and the "three-minute PhD" in the academic environment. These are all examples of explaining and communicating new innovative and exciting information in as few words as possible to an individual, who may or may not know you and, thus may not be interested in your work.

5.8 STAY FOCUSED

You should know that you will suffer many setbacks. Despite the numerous setbacks you are likely to encounter as you probe deeper into your research project, stay on track, and focus on your work, so you can continue to search for a solution to your biological question. Setbacks and delays will arise for several reasons, many beyond your control. You should realize that they occur to all scientists. Analyze each setback and identify what you can learn from it so that you can continue to move forward and remain well focused on your research objectives. By sticking to solving the problem, there often is a payoff. It may be an awesome payoff. It is exciting to discover something new, be it a new gene/protein, a new cellular metabolic or signaling pathway, a new concept on how a disease progresses, and/or a new cell function.

5.9 ACHIEVING RESILIENCE

Training to become a life science/biomedical researcher is likely to result in emotionally demanding periods of stress for you. You will need to be aware of these and deal with both inevitable stress that unfortunately is part of the job as well as unnecessary stress that you can eliminate by changing your own behavior.

Learn to Deal with Internal and External Generated Stress

In inevitable stressful situations, your goal is to learn to cope with them. You will feel the strain of external demands that impact on you and that you are expected to handle in a positive and successful way. These will include the standard stresses of course work, e.g., assignment deadlines, examinations; entering a new research environment, as transitions involved in your stage of training are stressful, demanding work-loads, developing a rapport with your supervisor, meeting milestones and preparing for student advisory committee meetings.

Serious unnecessary stresses will occur if you are not aware of milestones and not clear on the expectations of your own supervisor and those of the program. Once you have accurate information, you should be able to eliminate the stress by understanding what the milestones and expectations are. Then you can plan on how to achieve them.

There are also internally generated stresses which may interfere with your progress in your program. These include your own lack of confidence in your ability to carry out your research work; your over-reactions to difficulties and failures in your experimental laboratory work; your feeling that you are falling behind in your knowledge of the current literature; your perceived poor integration into the social and cultural fabric of your laboratory group and your department; feeling isolated and alone with no one to share your concerns and feelings with.

You will need to become resilient so that you will be able to resist adversity both real and perceived, without developing psychological, social, or physical disabilities that will impede your training. Resiliency is defined and characterized in many ways. One useful way is to consider resiliency as the ability to develop coping skills to reduce stress when you anticipate stress will occur. Another complimentary approach to define resiliency is the ability to develop your own personal characteristics and behavioral strategies to deal with stress once it occurs—the ability to bounce back quickly and effectively. You may attempt to change the situation to reduce stress or to avoid it completely. This, however, is not always possible.

Your graduate training environment should be a culture that nurtures resilience and well-being. As well, personal self-reflection is very useful in building your resilience by recognizing your own strengths and weaknesses and

Resilience Can Be Learned

thus, helping you to develop coping skills to reduce stress in the face of adversity. Resilience includes the ability to withstand adverse events and to bounce back effectively from adversity once it is experienced or even while it is occurring. In the latter case, you will continue onward despite the adversity that confronts you.

Resilience requires that you be well informed about your environment, understand what is expected of you, and know what are likely to be adverse situations and stumbling blocks that you will encounter. If you are aware that what you see as an adverse situation is in truth the norm for the activity, you will be able to cope much better. If you understand that procedural errors will occur as you learn new techniques and procedure, you will be better prepared to reduce their occurrence and should they happen, to cope with them.

Healthy living including adequate sleep, proper food nutrition, and exercise improves resiliency. Family and friends and out of laboratory social and leisure activities will provide a much better life–work balance and improve your resilience. Mindfulness-based stress reduction programs have become popular of late, and you should seek information about these types of programs to see if they will be of benefit to you. These programs provide training in self-regulation to reduce stress and manage emotion.

In matters related to stress and resilience, you may need some professional assistance to help you improve your resilience and mitigate stress. Do not hesitate to use appropriate university resources to enable you to continue to achieve your educational goals. When stress begins to impede your work and affects your psychological well-being, you need to seek professional assistance.

5.10 HANDLING FAILURE

Failures will occur in your research program and should be viewed as part of the norm for scientific investigations. Failures can occur at several steps in your research. You may realize that your idea or hypothesis may not be sound. It is based on an

| Accept and Learn from Failures |

incorrect interpretation of the literature or it is poorly conceived to allow you to move the science forward. Your technical skills must be of the highest quality or else your data will be meaningless. Despite careful work on your part, you may still run into a variety of design and technical problems that may prevent you from carrying out your experiments in a satisfactory manner. For example, in tissue culture your cells do not tolerate the protocols you wish to put them through although you may have made numerous modifications, and now you have to further redesign your experiments. You may interpret your findings incorrectly and move forward in an inappropriate manner to the next set of experiments. You cannot avoid failures but you can reduce the number of failures by discussing your planned experiments with supervisors, colleagues and technical staff, and by presenting frequently to your laboratory group to get useful immediate feedback. To avoid failure with techniques and instead to become proficient at specific technical skills, especially those not being used in your own laboratory, you may need to seek advice and visit a laboratory that has the technique up and running well. These experts can provide you with tips that you will never read about in any materials and methods descriptions in a published paper. This approach will prevent you from losing precious time as you carry out your experiments.

Despite working hard and seeking appropriate consultations from supervisors, peers, and experts, you may unfortunately find that you must abandon your project. Once it is obvious that the project cannot move forward, it is very wise to cut your losses and move on to another element of the project or even to a new project. Remember that scientific discovery is hard and unpredictable.

Failures can be more personal and may have a profound effect on you. The most difficult failure to face is leaving your graduate program without completing it and thus not obtaining your degree. If this happens very early on in your program then you end up losing some time, but you gain by not being trapped in a program that you are not succeeding in or have lost interest in and are no longer finding enjoyable and fun.

> Seek Guidance Quickly to Resolve Your Problems

This is not a failure, but more so a well thought-out change in interest and direction. However, if this happens late in the program, you may look at this as a failure to perform and you may be quite discouraged. Do not let your feelings smolder. As soon as you feel you are losing motivation speak openly to your supervisor, graduate coordinator, and/or mentor. Speaking to faculty may uncover other problems that, if corrected, would get you on track once again. This may help you resolve your initial problem quickly. Often graduate students have very high expectations of success and expect the success to occur rapidly. Unfortunately this is not how life sciences and biomedical research works. Instead there are many failed experiments, hard to explain outcomes, technical problems, and poor experimental design. Students become disillusioned and do not see a good return on all their hard work. Knowing and understanding how research projects evolve and that your experiences are not unique may help you to appreciate the difficulties in science and accept them. However, if you are truly unhappy and are rapidly losing interest, then you have to make an informed choice. Stick it out and finish your degree as best you can or cut your perceived losses and resign from your program. You do not want to do poorly and end up being terminated from your program due to consistent failure to meet the standards of your program. If you have been making careful informed decisions along your pathway, it is unlikely that you will find yourself in this predicament. However, there is no guarantee that it will not occur.

Can you switch supervisors to someone in your own department or in another department or program at your institution? Yes, you can if you meet all the conditions in your department/institution. First you must speak to your graduate coordinator (or equivalent) to seek advice on whether this is an appropriate option for you, and if so, how to achieve a switch. You need to consider new projects and new supervisors very carefully since the same issues may come up again in a new setting. You do not want to find out that the grass is not greener on the other side of the fence. You need to seriously consider whether a change in scenery will solve your difficulties or whether it is best for you to take a break and/or consider a different pathway. If you switch, be aware of time lost in your program and make sure that there is student stipend funding in place in your new setting.

5.11 LEARNING TO FACE REJECTION

Graduate students find rejection hard to handle. Following failures and rejections, you need to bounce back. You need to understand that failure and rejection are part of the "game" of science, which can nevertheless be harsh.

In life sciences, the two common areas of rejection that you are likely to face are rejection of a manuscript submitted to a journal and rejection of a scholarship application submitted to fund your scholarship/stipend. It is rare to have a manuscript accepted as is without any modification. The journal rejections are always accompanied by reasons for rejection written by the journal reviewers and the editor. Usually there is no reason given if your scholarship application is rejected. You have to learn how to read these critiques, often with the help of mentors and colleagues, to assess whether the paper just needs minor changes or whether major modifications are required before resubmission. The latter may need more experiments which could take up to a year or more to complete. You also need to make sure there are no fatal flaws in your manuscript or proposal which cannot be overcome by modifications. In this case, you may need to make very major changes which may alter the project drastically or even actually abandon the project and start over. You do have an opportunity to communicate with the editor of the journal if you feel you were unjustly treated. The editor has the final say and will let you know if she feels your complaints merit further examination. However, as a resilient scientist, you will learn from setbacks and make the required changes that will propel you forward to success. The key is to carefully regard the criticism and determine how you can benefit from the advice.

You should carefully review your rejection for a scholarship or studentship. Find out if you may reapply in the next competition and then consult with your supervisor, mentor, and your peers, especially those who have been successful, on how you can improve your application to be more competitive the next time around.

Coupled with failures and rejection, there are successes. Be sure to celebrate your successes, especially with peers, friends, and family. We tend to dwell on the rejections and failures, but we should focus foremost on our successes. Laboratory groups celebrate a successful thesis defense, publication of a manuscript, receipt of an operating or equipment grant, and receipt of studentship and scholarship awards. On a more personal level, some laboratories have a fine tradition of celebrating birthdays and special holiday events. These celebrations strengthen the laboratory group as a community of scientists and provide you with models on how to build your own successful research groups when the time comes.

Independence in a Protected Environment

CHAPTER 6

Postgraduate Studies: Preparing to Launch

6.1 CHOOSING A POSTDOCTORAL POSITION

6.2 YOUR POSTDOCTORAL CAREER DEVELOPMENT PLAN

6.3 HOW TO ACHIEVE POSTDOCTORAL SUCCESS

6.4 LEARNING MANAGEMENT AND THE BUSINESS OF SCIENCE

6.5 UNDERSTANDING MANUSCRIPT AND GRANT REVIEW

SUMMARY

The outcome of your postdoctoral research will have a significant impact on your future job prospects, so plan your postdoctoral position carefully. The search for an appropriate postdoctoral position can be a long process; therefore, you should begin your search well in advance of completing your PhD, at least a year to eighteen months beforehand. You must be well informed when you select a postdoctoral position. You need to feel that there is a good fit between you and your supervisor. You need a productive laboratory that is working on important problems. Postdoctoral education will allow you to learn new techniques and disciplines which will enhance your current graduate knowledge base. A postdoctoral position is designed to have you carry out high-quality research with very little supervision and to publish in high-impact journals. Thus an important consideration is to find out how much independence you will have. Little independence will not do you well. As a postdoctoral trainee, work on improving communication skills and build scientific networks with other researchers to expand your prospects for your future job. Pay close attention to progress in your research project since you have limited time to produce high-impact work. Be sure to learn how to manage and operate a research laboratory and how to review scientific manuscripts and research grants while you are still in your postdoctoral training environment. This will make the transition to running your own laboratory much easier.

Planning for a Career in Biomedical and Life Sciences. DOI: https://doi.org/10.1016/B978-0-12-814978-2.00006-5

Make sure to utilize your Postdoctoral Career Development Plan effectively by paying attention to achieving competencies and milestones. If your plans change and you decide to prepare for nonacademic positions, make sure that during your postdoctoral studies you begin to acquire excellent professional skills and comprehensive information on these other careers that you are considering. A Postdoctoral Career Development Plan should be used to guide your current research milestones and competencies as well as to explore alternate careers.

6.1 CHOOSING A POSTDOCTORAL POSITION

You should have been exploring postdoctoral positions well in advance of completing your PhD training. If you plan to consider academia especially at research intensive institutions and universities and even certain industry positions, postdoctoral training is almost universally required. You should plan to carry out your postdoc in the best place possible, preferably where there are strong research clusters of several investigators in your field. You may wish to interview with several possible advisors within the cluster to identify a best fit for your needs. You also need to make sure that the location will provide a fine quality of life for you and your family. Explore this carefully.

The search can take more than a year from preparation of application to landing the position. Popular laboratories fill up quickly and there may be waiting lists. Many positions are advertised in the fall, with interviews taking place in January to March. Initial contacts can be made in a variety of ways: at scientific meetings, and through visiting lecturers, job postings in journals and websites, word of mouth and networking, and other informal means. Your supervisor and other department members can be very helpful as well. Even if you are applying for a position at your current institution or at one you know well, treat it like an unknown entity because you are now looking at it through the lens of a postdoctoral applicant.

Keep your CV up to date. When citing an award, explain the award so that the reader will understand its importance. You should describe your role in any publications cited since they will often be multi-authored. When requesting a letter of reference, provide the referee with a draft letter to ensure they have all the factual details correct. They will edit the letter to reflect their own style of writing and add their evaluation.

6.2 YOUR POSTDOCTORAL CAREER DEVELOPMENT PLAN

Templates are now available for developing Postdoctoral Career Development Plans which you and your supervisor/advisor should complete and use as a dynamic guide to chart the course of your post-doctoral training (Box 6.1). Create milestones along your path to completion which are very beneficial and help you set the pace in the open-ended environment most postdoctoral trainees work in. Revisit the plan and the milestones frequently to make sure that you are on track (Box 6.1) and that you are achieving the required competencies to allow you to move on to your first job (Fig. 6.1).

> Postdoctoral Studies Require Clear Objectives and Goals to Achieve Success

---

Box 6.1 Postdoctoral Career Development Plan

Plans, Competencies, and Milestones

- The postdoctoral research career development plan is designed to identify competencies to be achieved and milestones to be reached during your postdoc.
- Begin to write the plan before you start your postdoctoral program and your research project(s). Discuss the plan with your postdoctoral supervisor.
- In comments, provide some details including outcomes.

Trainee Name:
Status:
Date Plan Initiated:

Postgraduate Training

Supervisor: Name
              Rank
              Department(s)

Mentor(s):   Name
              Rank
              Department(s)

Courses:

1. University
2. Non-degree or non-university

Research

Title of Project(s):

1. Why is your area of research important?
   Comment:
2. What gap in knowledge are you trying to fill?
   Comment:
3. How is your project original?
   Comment:
4. What research skills will be critical to the success of this project?
   Comment:
5. Which meetings/ conferences would be best suited for presentation of your project?
   Comment:
   a. Local
   b. Regional/ National
   c. International
6. What journal(s) in your field would be best for publishing your work, and why?
   Comment:

Research Qualifications and Certifications

Check the box if you have been exposed to and learned these skills and competencies

☐ **Code of Student Behavior**
   Comment:
☐ **General Standard Operating Procedures in Life Sciences Laboratory**
   Comment:
☐ **Laboratory Health and Safety**
   Comment:
☐ **Animal Care Course/Procedures (as applicable)**
   Comment:
☐ **Human Research Ethics Training (as applicable)**
   Comment:
☐ **Research Integrity Training**
   Comment:

Research Skills and Competencies
☐ **Critical Reading of Literature**
   Comment:
☐ **Experimental Design**
   Comment:
☐ **Technical Skills**
   Comment:

☐ **Analysis and Interpretation of Research Findings**
Comment:
☐ **Aid Supervisor in Journal Manuscripts/Grant Reviews**
Comment:
☐ **Entrepreneurial Skills**
Comment:
☐ **Laboratory Management**
Comment:
☐ **Leadership Skills**
Comment:

Dissemination of Research Results
☐ **Informal Communication of Research**
    ☐ To Supervisor
    Comment:
    ☐ To Laboratory Group
    Comment:
    ☐ To Other Laboratories and Fellow Students in the Program
    Comment:
☐ **Poster Presentations**
    ☐ Local/Away (e.g., Scientific Meeting)
    Comment:
☐ **Oral Presentations**
    ☐ Local/Away (e.g., Scientific Meeting)
    Comment:
☐ **Writing Scientific Report or Abstract**
Comment:
☐ **Writing Manuscript for Publication**
Comment:
☐ **Elevator Pitch**
Comment:

Noncurricular and Extracurricular Activities
☐ **Department/University/Hospital Student Groups**
Comment:
☐ **Outreach Programs (e.g., tutoring, mentorship)**
Comment:
☐ **Personal Activities at University or elsewhere**
    ☐ Sports
    Comment:
    ☐ Arts/Music
    Comment:
    ☐ Hobbies
    Comment:
    ☐ Other
    Comment:

Preparing for Job Market
- [ ] **Career Planning Lectures/Seminars (List those attended)**
  Comment:
- [ ] **Networking/ Important Contacts**
  Comment:
- [ ] **Postdoctoral Professional Development**
- [ ] **Job Hunting, Curriculum Vitae, Interview Skills**
- [ ] **Exploring Academic Job Opportunities**
  Comment:
- [ ] **Exploring Nonacademic (private, public sector, not-for-profit) Job Opportunities**
  Comment:
- [ ] **Short Internships**

Next Steps
- [ ] Applying for Academic/Private/Public Sector/Not-for-Profit Jobs

6.3 HOW TO ACHIEVE POSTDOCTORAL SUCCESS

The postdoc in biomedical and life sciences provides you with three important opportunities. First you learn new techniques and disciplines which will expand your knowledge base and your research expertise. Second, you will have the opportunity to carry out independent research work with very little supervision. You are still in a protected research environment but you can be highly innovative on your own. Take ownership of your project and become the world expert on the problem you are working on. This prepares you for a career as an independent investigator. Third, you should be able to produce excel-

Show Independence

lent work. You will be able to present this work at scientific meetings, a process that will allow you to meet and discuss your work with investigators in your field. Smaller meetings are most desirable since you will have a much better opportunity to meet like-minded scientists. These folks may be very helpful to you as you begin to explore permanent job opportunities. Also apply for presentation awards for these meetings. Your research should result in high-impact first authored publications. These are critical in competing successfully for academic positions, especially at research-intensive universities. Industry also appreciates well-published researchers. During the latter stages of your postdoctoral studies, some institutions allow for postdocs to apply for postdoc-to-faculty transition grants where these are available. These are extremely useful in facilitating your transition to a faculty position, so explore these opportunities carefully.

6.4 LEARNING MANAGEMENT AND THE BUSINESS OF SCIENCE

During your postdoctoral research, you should be actively learning how to operate and manage an independent laboratory. Learn the essential components of laboratory management and feel free to ask questions especially from laboratory managers, supervisors, and senior scientists to clarify issues. There is usually no formal course to do this, so most of the time you are left to learn on your own. In a large research laboratory, laboratory management may be done for you by the laboratory manager, so you may not actively consider or participate in it. However, once you are required to build and manage a science team on your own, you will regret not having paid close attention while you were in training. In the near future, it is likely that more graduate and/or postgraduate programs may include formal instruction on laboratory management including financial planning, budgets, human resources, and team building.

| Learn the Business of Science |

6.5 UNDERSTANDING MANUSCRIPT AND GRANT REVIEW

If you have not had these experiences as a graduate student, it is now important to learn how to review scientific manuscripts and research grant applications. To do this, ask your supervisor if you can help her on these tasks. If you learn how these are critiqued by reviewers, you will be able to improve your own manuscript and grant writing.

You can discuss the different templates that different journals use to guide reviewers in their review. This will give you an idea of what the editor and the editorial board are looking for in a manuscript. Each journal has a statement describing the types of studies they publish, that is, the field or discipline of study and/or the techniques their readership is interested in. This defines the aim and the scope of the journal. For example, there are many journals that publish in the area of cardiovascular science and medicine. Some may focus on the heart or on blood vessels or both, with an emphasis on basic science, translational, and/or clinical studies. Some may be disease-oriented, publishing on atherosclerosis, lipids, or transplantation. Others may focus on biomedical conditions such as heart failure or congenital heart disease. You will learn that the topic of your manuscript is a very important criterion in having your manuscript accepted for publication. A study may be excellent, but if it does not fit the stated scope of the journal, it will be rejected. You will also learn the criteria that editors ask

> Learn How to Review Journal Manuscripts to Improve Your Own Submissions

reviewers to rank the manuscript on, such as originality and quality of experimental design, execution, and data analysis. The editor will want you to comment on statistical analysis as well. The quality of figures and tables are also important in the review. The editor wants to know if there is new knowledge and the likely impact of the described discovery on the field and on science in general. If it is simply a rehash of work already in the literature, perhaps done in a different model, it is much less likely to be published in a quality journal. So when you review, you have to be familiar with the literature on the topic. Once your review is complete, you are usually asked to provide a recommendation for publication: Accept as is, Minor Modifications, Major Modifications, Reject with chance to resubmit, and Reject. If there is any suspicion of breach of scientific integrity, you must communicate this to the editor in your confidential response to the editor. Once you complete your review, you will compare notes with your supervisor and she will sign off on the review and send it to the journal editor. You will also learn that the process is confidential and you cannot utilize or communicate the contents of the manuscript to anyone. Your review is usually anonymous to the author(s) since you do not sign the "comments to the author." The confidential comments to the editor are made separately. Your anonymous "comments to the author" is submitted to describe your findings, to describe suggestions to improve the manuscript, and to provide reasons for your recommendation for publication. If you are suggesting modifications or a possible resubmission, the author(s) needs to know and understand what scientific concerns you have about the manuscript. In addition, many journals will send the "comments to authors" to all reviewers, usually two to three, so you may compare your review with others. This is solely for your own information. Although carrying out reviews is time consuming, you will benefit from this process.

To review grants, you need to read up on the agencies' procedures and rules for grant submission. There are clear instructions on the parameters for assessing the grant proposal. You may indeed use these parameters to frame your review. You need to explain why you perceive a given issue as a strength or a weakness of the proposal. It is important to convey what are serious concerns and flaws and what comments are meant to improve the grant. This should reflect your final scoring/rating of the proposal.

You should not review a submitted manuscript or a grant proposal if you have a real, or even a perceived, conflict of interest.

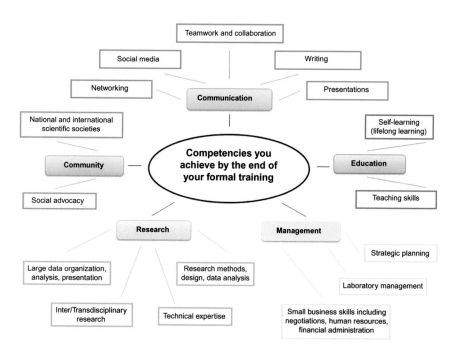

Figure 6.1 Competencies you achieve at the end of your formal training.

Life Continues But the Rules Are Different

CHAPTER 7

Your First Job: Choosing Well in Academia

SUMMARY

The search for a job is a long process. You should begin the process at least one year in advance of completing your training. Utilize word of mouth, networks, job sites, and advertisements in journals. Utilize informational inquiries where there is no position listed. Typically you will submit a well-organized curriculum vitae, an innovative research plan, and the names of referees who may be called upon to write reference letters. If you reach the search committee's short list, you will be invited to visit the institution. The search committee will assess your fit for the position and for the institution and department as a whole. Being very well informed about the department/institution shows your hosts that you are well prepared for the visit and serious about your intentions to work at the institution. Your scientific talk should be well rehearsed and well presented. Show yourself to be collegial and to function as a team player, since these are important selection criteria. Interviewing at a variety of institutions will help you to learn about the interview process

Planning for a Career in Biomedical and Life Sciences. DOI: https://doi.org/10.1016/B978-0-12-814978-2.00007-7

and allow you to see what other institutions are offering which will help your later negotiations. Follow up your visit with a thank you note to your hosts. If you are invited back for a second visit, be well informed when negotiating space, salary, benefits, and start-up packages to ensure that you are receiving the best offer possible to enable you to establish a successful research program. Do not rush to hire staff and trainees. Look for the best and be actively involved in the hiring process. These individuals will be doing much of the work in the laboratory; therefore, it is imperative that they are of high quality.

7.1 EXPLORING JOB PROSPECTS

You should explore job prospects well in advance of completing your training. The job search can take more than one year from preparation of applications to landing the job and negotiating the start-up package. Many academic positions are advertised in the fall, with interviews taking place in January through March. Initial contacts can be made in a variety of ways: at scientific meetings, meeting visiting lecturers, job postings in journals and websites, and through other informal means. Many successful candidates report that word of mouth and networking are very important avenues for finding out about job prospects. Your supervisor and other department members can be very helpful as well. Even if you are applying for a position at your current institution or at one you know well, treat it like an unknown entity. You now have to consider it from a faculty point of view and not from that of a trainee, which is a very different perspective. It does not hurt your cause to interview at several institutions so that you learn about the interview process and find out what each institution is offering. This is helpful in understanding how to rate an offer and how to frame your negotiations. Understand the market pressures so you can pursue appropriate negotiations. When selecting academic or industry opportunities, ensure that there is a culture of diversity, equality, and fairness present. At my own institution, candidates are informed in the job description that the university is "strongly committed to diversity within its community and especially welcomes applications from racialized persons/persons of colour, women, Indigenous/Aboriginal People of North America, persons with disabilities, LGBTQ persons and others who may contribute to the further diversification of ideas."

> Networking is an Effective Tool for Job Searching

7.2 ACADEMIC JOB DESCRIPTION

A faculty position as an independent investigator generally means that you have been assigned laboratory space in your institution to set up a research laboratory. An academic position may have different conditions. It may be tenure track/tenure, limited contract, limited contract with opportunities for extension, or some combination of these. Some positions are contingent on you having external support, full or partial, for your salary. You decide on your research program, plan it, and obtain funding for it. You hire technical and scientific staff and you supervise and mentor undergraduate, graduate, and postgraduate students. Independent does not mean that you do not collaborate or work with teams and in networks of scientists. Team-based research is very important in the biomedical and life science research of today, and does attract considerable funding to tackle important questions, often of a global nature.

7.3 PREPARING YOUR ACADEMIC APPLICATION

When you apply for a position, provide a professional looking CV that is clear and unambiguous. Remember the search committee will be receiving many applications to review. Identify your role in publications, especially multi-authored ones. Do not mix abstracts with publications. List chapters, books, and other non-peer-reviewed articles separately. Present a well thought-out research plan that is not too long but is innovative in nature and feasible at the institute to which you are applying. If you are carrying out basic discovery research, consider how your discoveries may be translated if this is appropriate. Translation that leads to commercialization should be considered as well. You should obtain feedback from colleagues and mentors before submitting your research plan. You should have had a frank discussion with your current supervisor about which projects you can take with you when you leave her laboratory. You do not want to compete directly with your postdoctoral supervisor. You need a research program that is your own. Keeping in contact with a former supervisor is to be encouraged, and even collaborating is fine, but you need to show research independence.

> Your Research Plan Must Be Well Developed

7.4 HOW TO SELECT REFEREES

You should pay attention to choosing appropriate referees. You should let your referees know beforehand that they may be contacted. Send them a CV and research plan so they understand your current situation and future plans. Referees should know you well. They should be able to provide critical analysis of your work and describe how you work in a group. Collegiality is an important feature in choosing both faculty for departments and investigators for industry. If an individual hesitates when you ask for a reference, do not use them as a referee. Search committees do expect to see letters from those who know you best, e.g., supervisors and former employers. If these are absent, you need to explain why.

7.5 ASSESSING TEACHING

If you have teaching experience, this is a plus but, in many cases, teaching experience may be limited during your training period. However, you will present a seminar, so search committees and interested faculty and students will be able to view your organizational and presentation skills firsthand, and see how you handle a discussion of your work during the question period. It is essential that you adhere to your assigned time and leave time for questions from the audience. The seminar provides some information to your hosts about your teaching potential. Make sure you bring the appropriate format to present your talk so as to avoid a technical problem arising during the presentation. Find out if your seminar will be transmitted to other locations, and if so, format your talk appropriately. Ask to check the AV equipment beforehand. Many universities require candidates to do a chalk talk in addition to giving a formal seminar; so prepare for this as well.

7.6 HOW TO BEHAVE ON YOUR INTERVIEW VISIT

An essential objective of your interview is for you to articulate what you want your job description to be. It is useful to have it written down in your own notes. Know where you can be flexible and where you cannot. A tactic to be avoided is to modify your job description during your interviews to suit the need of

> Be Well Informed About The Institutions You Interview At.

the institution. This is not useful since it calls into question your motivation. An attitude that conveys the notion that "I will do anything to get a job at your institution" is not a strong selling point at all.

Know as much as you can about the department you visit and the overall institution as well. Review websites. Be familiar with the research that is ongoing and know who is doing what. Know what the priority programs are in the department and at the institution. Identify potential collaborators before your visit by reviewing information on the departmental and institutional websites. Know who you will meet and review their work and publications. Learn about how the institution handles intellectual property and commercialization of discoveries.

Even before you arrive, have a set of questions that you need answered on this first visit. Remember this is your first visit so not everything needs to be covered and specifics are not always necessary. Your main objective is to determine whether this is a suitable place for you to initiate and develop your career and to live in a safe and interesting location. The search committee has at least three important issues to explore with you. They need to decide if you have what it takes to set up an independent productive research program, if your program fits well with the department's research and teaching goals and objectives, and if you yourself will fit well into the collegial group of faculty in the department. Departments want to recruit team players with very good people skills. Show enthusiasm and demonstrate that you are very interested in the position. This is best conveyed by demonstrating that you are well prepared for your visit.

> Fit and Collegiality are Essential

7.7 LEARN TO NEGOTIATE EFFECTIVELY

Do not be shy to discuss salary, start-up packages, and space, but that can be done in general terms and often toward the end of your visit when both you and your potential Chair/Director feel more comfortable with each other. These discussions are best conducted in private with your Chair/Director, not in front of a search committee. Do see the space offered. You should have some notion of what you would like to have included in your start-up package.

> Think Carefully About Start-up Packages

The real negotiating usually occurs on your second visit when details become very important. Then you need to create and present a comprehensive budget for the first three to five years which will become your request for start-up funding. Include personnel salaries, laboratory and office equipment, material and supplies, student stipends, and support to travel to scientific meetings.

7.8 HOW TO MAKE THE BEST START-UP FUND PROPOSAL

It is important to make sure you have what you need to start your program and to work for at least three to five years without major external funding. You will provide the Chair or Director with a list of equipment that you need—either as your own or as communal infrastructure equipment to which you need unrestricted access. Indicate how frequent this access will be and ask what the user cost will be. Your start-up need not be constructed to achieve a specific dollar value. The total dollar value depends on what you need and should reflect the true costs at the specific institution. For example, salaries for technical and administrative support staff vary in different regions of the country and in different institutions. Many faculty members feel that they must obtain everything in their start-up package. You need to obtain what you require in order to launch your career successfully as noted above. Do not expect to be in the same position as a senior faculty who has been at the institution for a while and has amassed resources. Successful senior faculty have proven by deed and activity that they are worthy of further support from the department/institution. Thus if you are successful, there will be opportunities down the line and beyond your start-up package to obtain more resources. If you get the impression that your start-up package is your only opportunity, then you may wish to rethink whether the institution is a place for you to build and maintain your career beyond the initial start-up period.

Investigate external peer-reviewed granting opportunities from relevant agencies. Inquire about internal grant competitions. Is there formal support and mentorship for junior faculty when they apply for initial grant funding? Does the department offer internal peer review and/or grant editing services? Inquire about the possibility of internal scholarships or training grants for graduate students and postdocs. Often allocations of these scholarships may be negotiated into your initial contract.

7.9 SALARY AND BENEFITS NEED CAREFUL CONSIDERATION

To negotiate your salary, be well informed. Find out what the salary scale is at the institution. In many jurisdictions they are listed on public websites, especially if faculty are considered to be government employees. You may get this information from your faculty associations, human resources, and/or contacts in the current faculty. Understand the benefits that you are eligible for. This research will give you a sense of what salary package is reasonable. You may indicate that you were looking for a little more and explain why. You may also ask if there is any opportunity to take on additional responsibility that does attract extra salary. Also understand how your salary will grow over the years and how this impacts your pension plan. When you begin as a junior faculty, pensions seem far off; however, they are important for you and your family. Ask about coverage of moving costs and travel to your new position for you and your family, if applicable. Do not discuss specifics of your offer with future colleagues at your institution. Financial issues are sensitive and are best kept private.

> Be Well Informed When You Negotiate

7.10 HOW TO TRANSITION TO YOUR OWN LABORATORY

You should try to have enough infrastructure and supplies that you need on site to start your academic research program as soon as possible after you arrive. Setting up a functional laboratory usually takes longer than you expect. Waiting for laboratories to be built or renovated and equipment to arrive may delay you considerably. It is also a poor excuse for lack of productivity when applying for external research grant funding. Thus, finish as much work as you can in your postdoctoral laboratory so that publications will come out as you set up your own laboratory in the new facility. There may be some overlap as you wind down your postdoctoral position and begin your faculty position. You may find yourself commuting for a period of time. Clear this with your advisor and also ask if you may begin writing start-up types of grants before you leave your postdoctoral program.

7.11 SETTING UP YOUR OWN LABORATORY

You will use your start-up funds wisely to set up your laboratory. Cost out all expenses accurately. Review your budget for the first three to five years and make revisions as required. Make sure to include cost of inflation. Obtain correct personnel salary scales and include benefits. Renewal of existing institutional contracts may result in sudden increases in the salary of trainees and personnel while you are setting up. Understand who are the preferred vendors for your institution and check what discounts you can expect either through the institution or through your own direct negotiation with the sales people. Explore equipment prices carefully and clarify whether setup costs and training costs are included. Sometimes demonstration models are available at a discount. Meet your neighbors in your own department and also in other departments. Find out what they do and what types of equipment they currently have. You may be able to share large pieces of equipment with another laboratory, thus saving on precious start-up funds, or if colleagues also need the new equipment, you may wish to purchase it together.

> Take Great Care in Setting Up Your Laboratory

7.12 HIRING TRAINEES AND STAFF

Hire good people—do not rush hiring. Your students, postdocs, and technicians will be doing much of the work in the laboratory, so you must be able to attract excellent people who can help you achieve your scientific goals. Check CVs and obtain references. Interview all your candidates for employment and for training positions. You should always interview potential employees according to the procedures of your institution's Human Resources department. Students and postdocs should have track records that make them competitive when applying for scholarships and awards from external and internal sources. This is a very good benchmark for determining the quality of the student and usually reflects performance in academic courses, research experience, evidence of research productivity, and letters of reference. Initially, you will be the only one interviewing candidates. It is useful to ask an experienced colleague to assist you with the interview. Once there are students and staff in your laboratory, include them in the interview process. This is important since your existing laboratory personnel will have to work with the new hires. Often, your existing laboratory personnel are the best individuals to assess the fit and compatibility of candidates for your laboratory team.

> Hire High Quality Individuals for your Laboratory Team

Your Initial Employment Is Still Part of the Journey and Not Your Destination

CHAPTER 8

Your Next 10 Years: Tenure and Promotion

SUMMARY

Once you obtain an academic faculty position, you need to immediately begin planning the next steps which lead to your evaluation for tenure and/or promotion. You will need to be viewed as excellent by your tenure committee in your research and teaching accomplishments and show promise of future excellence. Be aware of and utilize department/institution pretenure guidelines to focus your academic work. Avoid being unfocused in your research program since you will need a body of work to show your outstanding impact in your field. Criteria for tenure will vary from institution to institution. You must be very familiar with the tenure process to understand the timelines and the requirements for a successful tenure application. Engage your chair/director and your mentors in the process to guide you in your academic choices so that you are managing your time well and are well prepared to go forward for tenure and promotion. Make sure you have retained all your

Planning for a Career in Biomedical and Life Sciences. DOI: https://doi.org/10.1016/B978-0-12-814978-2.00008-9

teaching evaluations and help your chair identify students who may be called upon to provide reference letters for teaching, supervision, and mentorship. Consider whom you would recommend from the best scholars in your field to act as external referees. Other referees are selected by your chair and by the departmental tenure/promotions committee. The committee will assess your research productivity, your success in funding, the research impact of your work, and the success of your teaching including research supervision and mentoring. Internal and external awards acknowledging your excellent research and teaching are useful since they provide the committee with validation of your academic record. Be a good academic citizen by working with the leadership of your department to enhance institutional research and teaching platforms. Take on administrative duties and be an advocate for life sciences but manage your time very carefully since your first priority for achieving tenure and promotion is both your research productivity and impact and your success in teaching.

8.1 ACHIEVING TENURE AND ACADEMIC PROMOTION

While each institution has its own tenure/promotion requirements, there are several general principles to remember in academia. First, acquire a very clear understanding of the tenure process and/or the promotion process at your institution. Read and understand the guidelines as soon as you begin your position (Box 8.1). It is too late to find out as you go up for tenure/promotion that you should have done this or that. The main goal is to achieve academic excellence in research and teaching and thus you should know and understand the criteria for academic excellence in your institution. Second, many academic institutions have mechanisms in place to evaluate your progress while in the tenure stream with a focus on research and teaching. Participate fully in these assessments. These evaluations will point out strengths as well as areas of weakness and provide useful strategies to improve your situation. There are likely to be obstacles blocking your way to achieving tenure in both teaching and research. These obstacles need to be recognized and overcome, and pitfalls need to be avoided as noted in this chapter.

8.2 HOW TO NAVIGATE YOUR ENVIRONMENT

Once you have secured your job, you need to understand your university environment to meet the next set of challenges as you begin your

Box 8.1 Tenure Preparation Plan

Name:

Department:

Rank:

You should review and understand the tenure criteria before you sign your employment contract, so you know that the tenure expectations can be met by the terms of the contract.

This plan should be set up as soon as you begin your academic position. It should be initiated in collaboration with your Chair (or delegate or your direct supervisor). The plan should be referred to frequently and updated and/or amended as required.

Date of Commencement of Position:

Interim Evaluation Dates to Assess Progress:

Deadline for Tenure Application Submission:

General Preparation:

☐ I will seek advice from colleagues and academic leadership to plan my tenure application process

☐ I have mentors

☐ I have attended tenure information seminars organized by the University/Division/Department

☐ I am very familiar with tenure criteria

☐ I am very familiar with the tenure application procedures including deadlines

☐ I have consulted with those faculty leadership who will organize my tenure application, usually departmental Chair or delegate

Teaching:

☐ I am fulfilling teaching criteria, e.g., undergraduate, graduate

☐ I am collecting teaching evaluations, both quantitative and qualitative

☐ I am correcting teaching deficiencies

☐ I can create lists of students and faculty who can assess my teaching

☐ I have had interim teaching assessments from departmental or other committees that carry this out in my institution

☐ I have quality education publications, if applicable

☐ I have course material, including hard copy and electronic, to provide as part of my tenure dossier

☐ I supervise graduate students, undergraduate students

☐ I participate in graduate student advisory committees

☐ I have a list of students who can provide a reference letter

Research:

☐ I have an active research laboratory

☐ I have research funding, especially external peer-reviewed grants

☐ I have high-quality peer-reviewed publications

☐ I am known widely nationally/internationally for my research work

☐ I have been invited to scientific meetings, universities, and/or research institutes to present my work

☐ I have trained and am training doctoral stream graduate students

☐ I have a list of graduate students/postdoctoral trainees who may be asked to provide referee letters

☐ I have a list of well-recognized national/international referees from distinguished academic institutions who are acknowledged experts in my field of study and are free of conflict to provide letters of evaluation of my academic achievements

journey to achieve excellence. It now becomes essential for you to become very familiar with the career milestones you need to reach as your academic career evolves to achieve tenure and promotion. You need to continue to have a dynamic career plan. Be well informed of various options available to you and learn how to achieve them as you progress through the ranks at your institution (Box 8.1).

Understanding your academic environment is essential to navigating the departmental and university bureaucracy and achieving your milestones to obtain tenure and promotion. Understand the position of those who provide leadership and how they can help you. In the academic environment, the running of teaching programs and the research infrastructure are of major importance, and the department Chair has ultimate oversight and responsibility for the success of these programs. As a junior faculty member, you need to appreciate your fiduciary responsibilities and those of your Chair and her administrative team. There are very distinct differences in the role the academic Chair plays at different institutions. In some, the Chair is a rotating job which is simply administrative and more of a caretaker position. In others, the departmental Chair is appointed after a thorough academic search to translate the university's academic mission of scholarly activity into an operational strategic plan to enhance academics through innovative transformative planning and execution. In clinical departments, as in my own discipline, the Chair may also be responsible for directing the operations of a teaching hospital clinical department. Be a team player and help create a winning departmental team.

Any help you can provide your Chair and the university administration is much appreciated. Do not become a high maintenance faculty member but instead work with the Chair to facilitate her own responsibilities. Finally there are the intangibles which each Chair brings to her position and these have to do with her leadership, vision, determination, and adherence to the academic mission. The challenges are numerous and your Chair will need to expend much time and energy to mold a successful department. Your contributions in both the development and successful implementation of strategic academic plans will be greatly appreciated and will benefit your career as well as those of your colleagues.

> Add Value to the Administration of your Department

8.3 THE VALUE OF SCIENTIFIC NETWORKING

You are not working in a vacuum, so know of and meet investigators in your field. You will rely on them for advice, collaborations, exchange visits, and postdoctoral applicants. They will be in a position, if free of conflict, to act as external advisors and external referees. Attend meetings, especially small meetings where it is much easier to meet your colleagues and discuss science. Social settings during a meeting are a very good venue to interact with colleagues. Promote your own trainee's ability to attend scientific meetings with you. It is a very good investment of your funds and will be viewed very favorably by grant review and tenure committees. Many meetings offer competitive trainee travel awards so have your students apply for these.

> Interact Well with Your Community of Scientists

8.4 NAVIGATING INSTITUTIONAL PRIORITIES

Even in your pretenure stage you need to understand how to navigate institutional priorities. You will often be confronted by the phrases "there is no space" and "there is no money." You can interpret these statements to mean your space need or your money need is not high enough on the priority list to merit consideration. Then the ball is back in your court, and you have to make a strong argument backed by quantitative and qualitative data to support your needs. This reminds me of a situation early in my career as a university faculty member. As part of my limited clinical practice, I had a small office which accommodated my needs for my consultation practice in cardiovascular pathology at one of our teaching hospitals. Our hospital department moved to a new space in the same institution and unfortunately there was no space for an office for me. I was to remain in my current office which was now outside the confines of my department and a distance from my colleagues in their new space. This was not satisfactory to me and defeated the purpose of my being embedded in the department to provide much needed clinical expertise. I tried several avenues to acquire appropriate space without success. The response was always that my need was recognized and legitimate, but that there was "no space." I then spoke to my University Chair and he communicated with the hospital and informed them that if "I did not have a place to hang my hat" in the new departmental space, he was removing me from the hospital and assigning me elsewhere. Within a few days I received space for an office in the department. I learned three lessons: (1) make a strong argument; (2) have supportive mentors; and (3) there is no such thing as NO when it comes to space and resources. It is all about priorities.

8.5 MANAGEMENT OF YOUR SERVICE ACTIVITIES

Some amount of service activity is required since everyone must pitch in to help administer the organization in which they work. However, excellence in research and teaching are required for tenure. Thus, as a junior faculty budget your time very carefully for service. If you are doing your share of administrative work in your department as a junior faculty member, do not hesitate to decline a request to serve on yet another committee but indicate that once your current time commitments change, you are willing to take on

Budget Your Time Carefully   new responsibilities. In the early years, focus your administrative roles both at your institution and externally on activities close to your research activity, e.g., graduate committees and scientific meeting program committees. While serving on committees, be an active member and provide constructive advice to support and build your department, institution, or association. This is appreciated by your colleagues and helps you actively participate in structuring the environment in which you work.

8.6 TEACHING ASSESSMENT

As you approach tenure/promotion, you should have done some teaching. This will depend on the teaching assignments in your department or program. The highest teaching level is sole course director of a course you designed or even one already established by others. Inspiring classroom teaching and curriculum development, especially utilizing innovative methodologies, are positive characteristics in a tenure dossier. Some faculty publish their innovative curriculum accomplishments in educational or discipline-specific journals. In some cases, the availability of course teaching may be limited in your department so you need to gain some teaching experience and an opportunity to be evaluated for teaching through other means. You can give some guest (invited) lectures in a course in another program. You provide teaching in your capacity as a graduate supervisor and as a member of a graduate student advisory committee. Mentoring graduate and undergraduate students also counts for teaching if done in a rigorous fashion with bonafide mentoring strategies informing the process and outcomes being recorded. Some institutions assess teaching by utilizing expert teachers to evaluate in-class teaching. The reports generated become part of the teaching dossier.

> **Continually Upgrade Your Teaching and Supervisory Skills**

As chair, I had a faculty member hired in a nontenured position to develop an independent research program at an affiliated research institute. He made it well known to me that he wanted to teach as well. We finally found him a few guest lectures and some supervision of graduate student seminars. This started him on the road to teaching undergraduate and graduate students which he combined with his successful research program. When he came up for promotion, his teaching dossier had the achievements needed for promotion, in addition to his excellent research.

Teaching dossiers require a comprehensive description of teaching activities with course number and title, number of hours taught, number of students, type of teaching, and most important, teaching evaluations. These include student evaluations which usually focus on the effectiveness of in-class teaching. Students will focus on the appropriateness of the course workload, the course evaluation processes, the clarity and organization of notes and lectures, the organization of the course as a whole, and your availability to handle questions and problems. They usually communicate with you electronically or otherwise by face to face meetings. They appreciate prompt replies. They also appreciate your prompt return of class assignments and midterm examinations. Student evaluations should be carefully considered by you because they provide useful feedback to give you an opportunity to improve your teaching if necessary. Make sure to collect student teaching and course evaluations after each course you teach. It is very difficult to reconstruct evaluations years after the fact.

You need to have attracted high-quality graduate students and post-doctoral fellows who have been productive in the laboratory. You should have also been a member of student advisory committees. Graduate students and postdoctoral trainees who provide referee letters often focus on the quality of your supervision and on your performance as a mentor. Your engagement with students as a member of a student advisory committee is important, and I have read student reference letters commenting on faculty performance in that capacity. In addition to student evaluations, some departments/institutions have faculty teaching committees that do an in-depth analysis of your teaching, visit classrooms, and view your teaching material. Innovation in course development and course presentation are accorded high marks in the assessment of your teaching. These programs will help you improve your teaching evaluation and get you ready to come forward with a strong teaching dossier for tenure and/or promotion.

8.7 ACHIEVING A SUCCESSFUL RESEARCH PROGRAM

First and foremost, protected time devoted to your own research enterprise is critical. At the research intensive institutions, the highest priority must be given to your research activities. You require that 75% of your time is dedicated to research to become a successful, independent, well-funded, and productive life sciences/biomedical investigator with an international reputation for excellence in research.

> Protected Time for Research

You must choose a research program which is innovative and which will lead to important new discoveries. "Me too" or "lateral type research" will not advance your career. You need to work on important problems, the solution of which will impact on your discipline and if you are lucky, in science in general. You need to choose a feasible project that is doable during your pretenure period. Once you choose your problem, stay focused. Do not hesitate to ask for help or even collaboration to complete your work. Be careful not to accept too many other projects that colleagues want your collaboration on. This will spread you too thin and you will not be able to devote enough time to your own project. Having a wonderful reputation as a collaborative colleague is fine but you need to show a strong independent focus to compete for tenure. On occasion, you may run into a situation in which you are carrying out your experiments on your main project which is progressing well and you discover something very interesting. Since you cannot do everything, you have a dilemma. Do you put this interesting and potentially very important finding to the side and risk someone else finding it, or do you change projects? With tenure looming, if you switch, you may not have enough high-quality science when your tenure clock rings. Of course, every situation like this will be different; however, it is best to discuss this with your mentors and others whose judgment you trust. This is clearly a good news/bad news story and you need to give it careful and thoughtful consideration.

> Strive for High Impact Publications

8.8 STRATEGIES FOR RESEARCH FUNDING

On the research side, to obtain tenure you should have been awarded peer-reviewed funding as a Principal Investigator usually from at least two funding sources and had renewals. Writing research grants is the most important activity you do. Start early to leave enough time to write a thoughtful innovative proposal. Seek input and review from colleagues to improve content and readability. Many institutions have various forms of assistance for grant writers. Use these effectively. Ask colleagues to share samples of their successful grants. Be aware that there are differences in requirements among different agencies, and the scoring systems may also vary, especially in the weighting of different components of the grant. Most scientists consider investigator-initiated operating grants as the cornerstone of a successful research program and an essential driver for new discoveries. Actively seeking collaborations and membership on teams and networks is also important; however, budget your time carefully so that you do not become overextended. Being a co-applicant on a multi-investigator program is indeed useful, but you must be very clear and transparent in showing how you are making a major contribution to the team. Being a principal investigator on consortium type projects is an excellent career choice and is likely to advance your science effectively and efficiently.

8.9 UNDERSTANDING UNIVERSITY–INDUSTRY COLLABORATIONS

Currently there is much interest in academic scientists collaborating with industry. Although these still remain two distinct cultures, as modern science progresses there are definite benefits in promoting these collaborations, for instance, bringing different expertise, technology, and funding to the scientific table to allow academic scientists to create new platforms to carry out innovative research. Often the focus is on translational and applied research but not at the exclusion of basic discovery research. Since governments are supporting innovation in biomedical and life sciences as an economic engine and as a way to provide high-quality cost-efficient health care, there are substantial funding opportunities for university-industry-partnered research. Government agencies in

> Understand the Benefits of University-Industry Partnerships for Your Research Programs

many jurisdictions have developed competitive funding mechanisms to provide research dollars to collaborative efforts between universities and/or research institutes and industry. The two cultures are learning how to work successfully with each other and cope with the administrative burden that often is associated with these collaborations. Both sides recognize this and are working on ways to ease these burdens and streamline the administrative and legal processes that are required for collaborative research to occur across organizations. Institutions are also ramping up their administrative capacity to help academics overcome the hurdles and reap the benefits from possible commercialization opportunities that research partnerships between academia and industry may provide.

8.10 HOW TO ESTABLISH SUCCESSFUL PRODUCTIVITY

Your research program may start off with a few more modest publications to show initial productivity and independence. However, you should have progressed to a stage that high-impact publications have been and are being accepted for publication. This is what is required for receiving tenure. Quality should be placed well ahead of quantity.

You should be establishing your name for a body of innovative high-impact work which attracts attention from your colleagues. Your publications should appear in the highest impact subspecialty and general biomedical and/or science journals. These should lead to invited lectures to national and international scientific meetings and to universities and institutes. Invited reviews in well-recognized journals also indicate your recognition in your field. Do not be tempted by flattering letters to write reviews in less than high-impact journals. These will count little in terms of your scientific productivity and take you away from important work.

As your reputation grows, you will become involved with research review as an external reviewer of manuscripts and/or grant proposals. The quality of the journals that you review for is important, so prioritize your reviews to high-impact journals and journals in your discipline or areas of research. You may, although this is much less likely, as a junior faculty be asked to serve as an internal reviewer on a grant review panel. Many folks feel you should wait for at least five years so that your own research program is well established. These review activities are time-consuming so you must budget your time very carefully. Not obtaining your own grant funding because you are too busy reviewing others is not a useful way to advance your career and will not help you achieve tenure.

8.11 APPLYING FOR MERIT AWARDS

You are encouraged to apply for and receive personnel awards. Early career awards are usually very competitive and are a confirmation of the high regard your peers have for you and your work. These awards are often meant to identify and support rising stars. Applications are usually a time-consuming process so focus on applying for those awards which you have a very good chance of receiving. Seek information about the application process so you understand how best to complete the forms and what the agency is looking for in its awardees. Seek advice from senior colleagues and from former award winners. As you progress in your academic career and you build your track record of excellence, consider seeking nominations for Teaching and/or Research Awards, either locally and/or outside your institution. These recognize your own contributions and

Personnel Awards Are Prestigious

also are acknowledged by your department, institutions, and/or scientific or professional society as an indication of the excellence of their faculty and/or members.

8.12 YOUR PROGRESS IN A RESEARCH INSTITUTE

You may have launched your career in a research institute which has less of a teaching focus than the university. You may be affiliated or cross-appointed to the university but your evaluations are primarily done by your institution. Such evaluations may be undertaken in a number of ways. Commonly evaluations are carried out after three and six years. Initially you may hold a junior/associate scientist rank, and after two successful reviews you may achieve a scientist rank. Some institutions have a further senior scientist rank for their most accomplished investigators. The science is critically evaluated by internal and external experts in your discipline, and the same criteria of research excellence as considered in the university tenure and promotion process are applied. Your roles at the institute as a collaborator and as a good administrative citizen are also seriously considered. Today, in an era where the value of transdisciplinary science is well recognized, your successful team efforts on some of the global problems that your institution focuses on are highly valued.

8.13 WHY ADVOCACY IS REQUIRED

As a scientist it is important that you disseminate your work to the lay public even as a junior faculty member. This knowledge transfer is important as it informs the public that you are doing essential work that has an impact on them and on the environment they live in. Often with curiosity-driven research, the value of the increase in knowledge and understanding of the world around you is not readily apparent. Since the impact may not be obvious, a clear message needs to be delivered

> Be an Honest and Effective Advocate for Scientific Research

to the public that fundamental discoveries pave the way for successful applied research. In many cases, the fundamental discoveries do not have an immediate application; however, they contribute to a knowledge base that will potentially lead to future clinical impact. Basic science research is indeed the primary fuel for translational research. An example would be those scientists who made seminal basic science discoveries in the field of thrombosis that led to the use of biologic drugs to break up blockages in blood vessels to prevent and/or reduce the complications of heart attacks and stroke. Try not to oversell your work, but instead be factual and honest in transmitting information to the public. Do not overpromise what science can deliver. This knowledge transfer should be part of an advocacy agenda that each scientist should be involved in.

Why advocacy? In our society, people are required to make decisions on how to prioritize public and even private spending. As a scientist you have an obligation to advocate for the best possible infrastructure, education, and research funding to support a high-quality life sciences enterprise. How do you do this? First you need to believe that advocacy is important and that you are willing to spend your own precious time on it. Then you need to acquire some skills in advocacy. Most scientists need to learn these skills because they are often not intuitive. Scientific societies often sponsor initiatives to train you, provide you with needed facts, and even organize encounters with governments and the lay public that you are encouraged to participate in. You need to know how and what to present to the lay public and to members of government and industry. "Keep it simple, clear, and honest" is the best piece of advice I received. I present myself as a trusted member of the scientific community who is willing to share and explain up-to-date scientific information for the benefit of the audience. I tell stories that reflect the excitement of scientific discovery that often may have direct impact on the community and on members in the audience. The lay public should be convinced that it is in their own best interest to support research and education in life sciences.

Teaching and Research Institutions Are Valuable Community Resources and Require Constant Care

CHAPTER *9*

The Institutional Challenge to Train and Support Academic Biomedical Scientists

9.1 INSTITUTIONAL EXCELLENCE

9.2 INSTITUTIONAL TEACHING

9.3 INSTITUTIONAL RESEARCH

SUMMARY

Departments and universities depend on their faculty to maintain their commitment to excellence. You will find it very rewarding to be a "good citizen" of your department/program, faculty, and institution. You should have a sense of pride and feel obligated to contribute to maintaining the well-being of the academic environment you live and work in. Creating excellent educational programs and acquiring state-of-the-art equipment and facilities will enhance your own academic success as well as that of your colleagues. Time is a precious commodity and must be managed with care; however, contributing your fair share to creating and maintaining a dynamic high-quality science enterprise is a priority as well. Be pleased to serve on committees that identify and solve problems and bring forward strategic innovative solutions to strengthen the academic life of your institution.

9.1 INSTITUTIONAL EXCELLENCE

Once you achieve tenure and promotion, you now have the obligation to help your institution maintain its excellent reputation. The expectation is that you will maintain your own excellence, continue to make significant contributions to life sciences and/or biomedicine, and continue to link your research to excellent teaching. To achieve this, your senior leaders in universities and scientific institutions advocate for and create high-quality environments to support your research and teaching. This will support an environment that retains the very best biomedical scientists to generate and transmit new knowledge to fellow

Planning for a Career in Biomedical and Life Sciences. DOI: https://doi.org/10.1016/B978-0-12-814978-2.00009-0

scientists, trainees, and clinicians, thus creating a culture of scientific excellence. As a faculty member, you need to help your academic institution maintain and grow its capacity for high-quality sustainable research. This allows you to train high-quality students in excellent programs that equip them to face their own futures in both academic and nonacademic life sciences.

> To Practice the Best Life Sciences/Biomedical Research Help Create a Stable High Quality Science Enterprise.

You should support your institution in maintaining an environment that rewards innovation, fosters the ability to unravel the mysteries of biology, and nurtures innovative and transformative research. You yourself need to participate and lead high-quality programs that provide unique training to study and understand normal biology and clinical disease. A stimulating intellectual environment with state-of-the-art resources and time dedicated to research is needed to support your productive growth, especially in the early stages of your career. Universities, teaching hospitals, affiliated research institutes, granting agencies (both private and governmental), and industrial partners need to be encouraged by you to actively support these academic initiatives, create capacity to train young life sciences and biomedical scientists, and to support you, their mentors.

9.2 INSTITUTIONAL TEACHING

Institutions should not neglect teaching. When planning their research agenda, it is not either or, but instead, each compliments the other and offers students a strong educational program. Your institution should offer innovative teachers the opportunities to be able to link teaching to research and to state-of-the-art knowledge and technology. You should have the opportunity to be able to carry out research in education and if you wish to do so, make this the primary focus of your own academic mission. Faculty development opportunities in teaching are very important in advancing the quality of teaching. High-quality information technology is essential to carry out first-class teaching to undergraduate, graduate, and postgraduate trainees. Your institution has to generate and use reliable data to demonstrate that your students are obtaining a quality education and you as a faculty member need to lead these evaluation exercises.

9.3 INSTITUTIONAL RESEARCH

You are more likely to attract significant resources and excellent faculty and students when your academic leaders have the vision to initiate and maintain programs that promote innovation and encourage transformative research. Research programs need to be frequently adjusted to provide the very best opportunities for faculty. Institutions that create infrastructure and opportunities for multidisciplinary research to address important biological and medical gaps in knowledge are successful in our scientific community. Institutions need to adjust their academic resources to reward academic scholarship in fundamental discovery and translational research. A culture of innovation will lead to high-impact productivity and to wide international recognition in academic life sciences and biomedicine. Institutions need to be allowed to think big and be strategic and flexible to achieve academic success.

Academic Leadership Is Tough and Rewarding

CHAPTER 10

Into the Future: So You Want to Be an Academic Leader

10.1 ACADEMIC LEADERSHIP

10.2 THE FACES OF LEADERSHIP

10.3 DELIVERING LEADERSHIP

10.4 HOW TO ACHIEVE EFFECTIVE COMMUNICATION

10.5 AVAILABILITY OF THE LEADER

10.6 HEALTH AND SAFETY

10.7 HANDLING URGENT SITUATIONS

SUMMARY

Once you have been awarded tenure, you must continue your excellent research and teaching. However, you may aspire to holding leadership positions in your department/institution. This requires planning to first obtain junior leadership positions to provide you with necessary skills to then move into senior positions. You need to maintain your academic standing and lead by example. As a leader, some of your time is spent for the betterment of your scientific community. You should be well aware of your scientific and institutional environment which is necessary to provide strategic leadership and take advantage of planned and unplanned opportunities. You must gain the confidence of your faculty and be an excellent communicator. Mentorship skills are an important asset in leadership. As you lead, you must be transparent and inclusive and assess how best to move your department forward, especially to handle change. The institution has processes that you should follow carefully and resources to help you with a variety of issues including those involving faculty, staff, and students.

10.1 ACADEMIC LEADERSHIP

Leadership is a very difficult job if done well. You are responsible for the well-being of the people and the institution that you are leading.

Planning for a Career in Biomedical and Life Sciences. DOI: https://doi.org/10.1016/B978-0-12-814978-2.00010-7

You should focus on innovative ideas that benefit the group and that can be implemented well without discord. You are not a caretaker. You are not a manager. Instead you have the honor and the privilege to work on behalf of your constituents to improve their academic life.

I found leadership to be more than just being a manager. Quality management is essential to provide a well-functioning department that interacts well with its partners at the university and, in a medical department, with the hospitals. Management of budgets, educational programs, human resources, tenure and promotion processes and faculty, student, and course evaluations are some of the areas that need excellent administrative/academic management. However, leadership is a different issue. Leadership requires a well-focused and articulated vision. A smart leader blends her own vision with that of the faculty to adopt a vision that everyone can buy into. As a junior faculty, participate in these processes since your future to some extent is being planned. In arriving at the final vision the partners in the vision will have to compromise and reach a consensus; however, there are academic issues which cannot be compromised, otherwise the academic mission will not survive. What should not be compromised? Quality and scholarship.

The best preparation to be an academic leader is for you to begin by playing lesser leadership roles so that you can learn the job under less demanding conditions. Declare your interest in leadership. Current leaders should then be identifying you as interested in academic leadership. You will be groomed for local succession or for export to take on leadership elsewhere. Mentorship from established

Plan for Leadership Succession

leaders is extremely useful. You will need some administrative university experience, usually initially directing and managing a departmental program, e.g., Vice Chair education or research or graduate training. Chairs may move from smaller institutions where they "got their feet wet" to larger more complex departments in large institutions.

Learning on the job used to be the way it was done. Today the complexities of the job and the numerous oversight bodies and regulatory issues that exist require that academic institutions offer a curriculum for new administrative faculty, which is compulsory to complete successfully. In addition, you will benefit from taking advanced courses on university administrative management. You also need a mentorship structure in place once you secure the job, especially in the first months on the job.

Conflict of interest is an especially important concept to be aware of for leaders. Generally, a conflict of interest exists when current or even past relationships exist that influence or have the potential to influence professional judgments, decisions, or actions. The perception that a conflict of interest exists is also an important consideration to deal with.

> Avoid Conflict of Interest

10.2 THE FACES OF LEADERSHIP

Competent leadership in the academic setting has an external and an internal face. Externally, you as the leader need to be seen as the leader by the external community and as the spokesperson for the department if you are departmental Chair or for the division if you are Dean. You need to be well known externally and to be well connected with those who may interact with the department. Where your department/division needs to be represented, you as the leader should be there. Leadership by delegation of duties may send a negative message at many levels to the external community. You need to understand what may be delegated and what may not be. It is important that a unified message be presented that reflects department thinking rather than a diffuse and sometimes confusing message from a collection of delegates that you send to committee meetings. You need to get out a clear message, describing where you stand as a department/division on academic issues.

> Leadership Requires your Attention and Presence

The internal face is directed at the important relationships that are built up within the department/division. The faculty, staff and students need to know that the leader is there for them. If there is a problem, there is an open door, a confidential setting for frank discussion, and a readiness to provide useful advice. Clear communication that is forthright and honest creates this internal leadership. This leadership requires sensitivity, an understanding of human nature, and a willingness to spend time to guide and help those in your department/division. This same internal face sets the guidelines, the academic bar, and the accountability framework under which the department/division operates. Sometimes these may appear to be harsh; however, they should be fair, sensible, and put into place without creating internal conflicts that damage the fabric of the department/division. Wide consultation and town hall type meetings that explain the reasons for new regulations and changes are very helpful for a smooth implementation.

10.3 DELIVERING LEADERSHIP

There is no optimum style; you will develop your own. You can initially take a hands on approach so that you learn about how things work in your office or department and then delegate some authority to your administrative staff and designated colleagues as you see fit. There is no substitute for understanding the complexities of the job and being able to make informed decisions. The "hit and miss" form of decision-making is just that. It is unfortunate when the "miss" involves a major issue and you end up with a problem that is bigger than it originally was.

As an efficient and dedicated leader, you should begin by being hands on, and as staff and colleagues work with you, delegate more. The leader, however, should always be in the loop. Faculty and staff should understand that you need to know about current problems and about potential problems. It is very embarrassing and potentially harmful to the department if the first time you hear about something happening in your department/division is from an outsider.

Here are the paradigms most useful to you to become facile with (1) have a vision; (2) embrace innovation and change as required; (3) understand, consult, make a decision, and communicate; (4) assess risk; and (5) plan strategically so that you succeed in positioning your department well for the future.

10.4 HOW TO ACHIEVE EFFECTIVE COMMUNICATION

Being an effective communicator is a critical skill for leaders to have. Committee meetings should be as brief as possible and not run over-time ever. Always end on time, or even early if possible. Folks will appreciate that you value their time. You should however not prevent or inhibit useful discussion, and there should be sufficient time to hear all opinions. These opinions should be valued and never dismissed in an offhand manner. If you need to rebut on a critical issue, do it immediately in an even-handed way. Shouting and table banging are not useful in the academic community, nor is ridiculing the speaker.

Face-to-face one-on-one meetings are essential in dealing with faculty. Often you will gain valuable insight into matters by having frank discussions with your faculty members. It is reasonable to keep your one-on-one meetings short and make sure everyone knows this. Thus folks know you will give them your undivided attention but for a set period of time.

> Be Clear and Precise in All Communications

There should be mechanisms in the department to deliver clear, concise policy information that has been approved through the appropriate institutional governance. A new policy must be communicated to all concerned and should not be a surprise to your faculty since there has been appropriate consultation beforehand. A policy also requires an easily accessible implementation document which describes how to implement it.

10.5 AVAILABILITY OF THE LEADER

Unfortunately you cannot hide today and you will usually be in reach electronically. However, you should have a group of senior faculty to whom you can sign out to who are familiar enough with day-to-day items to handle them or more importantly decide what can wait and what needs your urgent and immediate attention. An administrative manager who has broad knowledge of the operations of the department is a good person to act as a point person and a filter when you are away. When you are absent from the university, you must inform those to whom you report to as well as key leadership colleagues.

10.6 HEALTH AND SAFETY

As a leader, you have a responsibility to ensure that occupational health and safety protocols and procedures are known and followed by all. Safety should be a major focus of the organization and you should provide the leadership to eliminate preventable harm. A review of security is important for both the administrative offices and for the offices and laboratories occupied by faculty and students. Universities and the hospitals have regulations, guidelines, and resources; however, as a leader, you have the responsibility to ensure that the guidelines are made clear, understood, and adhered to. In many institutions, your departmental health and safety status is routinely audited and infringements are flagged for correction.

10.7 HANDLING URGENT SITUATIONS

You should leave time in your daily calendar to be able to see someone within 24 hours. Your assistant should be able to assess urgency and oftentimes prevent a difficulty from becoming a catastrophe. A more comprehensive meeting if required could then be scheduled later at everyone's convenience.

At the meeting, find out exactly what the problem is and what the individual wants you to do about it. Often people just want to inform you about their situation, but they do not want you to get involved. Assure the individual that whatever they wish to keep confidential will be kept confidential. Sometimes you need to let the individual know that you must consult others for advice. Sometimes your assessment suggests that safety may be an issue and you must act for the common good. Let the individual know what you plan to do.

Ask if you can take notes and do so. At the end of the meeting, you should write down the action items that you and your faculty, student, or staff agreed to follow. Make sure they understand these very well. Place timelines on all the activities. Sometimes the institution itself has very specific timelines that must be followed. Make sure you are well aware of the university and faculty policies concerning the issue under discussion. You yourself may need to consult with others to clarify policy. Also direct your visitor to pertinent policies as well. Sometimes the issue is not in your jurisdiction but you must guide the individual to the appropriate place to receive help. Do not handle issues that are not in your jurisdiction, even if you think you are being helpful.

If an individual wishes to make a complaint and expects you to take action, you need to receive a written complaint signed by the individual. This avoids any miscommunication and also allows the individual to crystallize their complaint. Anonymous complaints are not useful and are difficult to pursue. The complainant should be made fully aware, by you, of options available to them. They should also be reminded to consult any collective agreements, memorandum of agreements, guidelines for appropriate academic behavior, or any other pertinent institutional policies and documents. What may make sense to you and to your complainant may in fact be in contradiction to an agreement under which you operate. So be well informed.

Remember you have numerous knowledgeable individuals to consult with. Know and understand the various services the institution has at hand. These are usually staffed by professionals with experience, on safety and security, harassment, family and health services, and so forth. The best approach is to go up the reporting ladder (e.g., chain of command). You can seek advice with or without naming individuals so that confidentiality can be maintained.

Enjoy Your Initial Employment, the Platform for Launching Your Career

CHAPTER 11

Your First Job: Preparing and Choosing Well for Nonacademic Careers

11.1 HOW TO TRAIN FOR A NONACADEMIC CAREER

11.2 LIFE SCIENCES PLATFORM

11.3 JOB CHOICES

11.4 PLACEMENTS AND INTERNSHIPS

11.5 HEAD HUNTERS

11.6 ADVANCEMENT IN NONACADEMIC CAREERS

SUMMARY

You are fortunate that life scientists/biomedical researchers have many nonacademic career opportunities available in industry, business, and professional disciplines. Some will keep you at the laboratory bench as a research scientist. Others will require that you apply your scientific research knowledge to either a nonresearch field, such as science writing, high school teaching, or science policy, or to a nonscientific field such as finance, business development, law, or information management and others. There are also clinical jobs available in biomedical health care, such as diagnostic molecular genetics, clinical biochemistry, or microbiology. You may become well informed about these nonacademic jobs even while you are a graduate or postdoctoral trainee. Make appropriate inquiries to understand the required qualifications you need to work in your new field of interest. However, do not neglect your current graduate or postgraduate research; it is an important qualification which provides you with unique professional skills and a science knowledge base which is attractive to gain employment. Thus complete a high-quality thesis with high-impact publications. You may find that networking in both academic and nonacademic realms will help you with your job search, as many nonacademic positions are advertised through word of mouth. Internships, placements, and volunteering are good ways to gain relevant experience and to expand your professional networks. After you have acquired a position, be aware of how to make

Planning for a Career in Biomedical and Life Sciences. DOI: https://doi.org/10.1016/B978-0-12-814978-2.00011-9

yourself competitive for your next promotion. Maintain your networks and join scientific and industry societies to keep abreast of the changes and opportunities occurring in your discipline.

A degree in biomedical and life sciences opens you up to job opportunities that exist outside of traditional academia. Many of you will pursue this nonacademic route since only about 15% on average of PhD graduates end up in academia. There are many nonacademic careers out there and being well informed about them is crucial to selecting a path to pursue (Fig. 11.1).

How do you prepare for a nonacademic job? There is no formula for doing this. Some nonacademic jobs require that you be job-ready, i.e., well-trained for the position, while other employers are willing to spend resources and time to train you. A graduate degree in biomedical and life sciences is an asset for some nonacademic positions and is essential for others. In fact, it is your scientific graduate training that will play a large part in shaping your nonacademic career. These

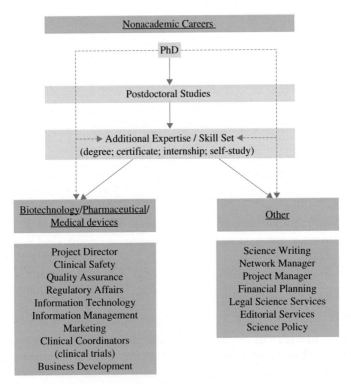

Figure 11.1 Nonacademic careers.

nonacademic careers are very heterogeneous in scope when compared to one another; however, in general, recruiters are looking for highly qualified applicants and so competition is stiff.

The same general principles discussed above in the context of academic apply to nonacademic training and job searches. An important qualification for nonacademic jobs includes a sound academic record which allows the recruiter to evaluate how you solve problems, write reports, and communicate. People skills and being a strong team player are very valuable assets and cannot be overemphasized. Recruiters will assess you on your abilities to work on teams with diverse perspectives in order to generate innovative solutions to the problems they work on. The postdoc or postdoc equivalent will still give you an edge in competing for jobs, especially the very good ones. Most employers will do reference checks focusing on your work ethic, compatibility with peers, management and communication skills, and your strengths and weaknesses related to your job performance. Always use social media responsibly since digital information cannot be contained and tends to live on for a very long time.

11.1 HOW TO TRAIN FOR A NONACADEMIC CAREER

In planning ahead, there are two important issues for you to consider. First, be very well informed about what is required to work in the nonacademic field of your choosing, including certification, licensure, and an internship, and learn about what training opportunities are available. Second, do not let your preparation for a complimentary or new career interfere with completing a strong biomedical/life sciences graduate degree, even though your interest is in the nonacademic world.

It is useful to begin exploring the new careers you are interested in while completing your degree. This will depend on how hard you want to work and how well you multitask. Do you just wish to explore career opportunities or have you already decided and wish to begin to prepare for your new career while finishing your current degree? Whether your plan is feasible is based on the demands of your current degree program and the requirements for training in your new area as well. Some life sciences programs do offer combined or dual graduate degrees/programs and/or opportunities for certification while completing your traditional graduate degree.

We often think of training as taking formal courses. With new emerging educational technologies, it is easier to gain access to knowledge. Independent learning is easier to do as education moves online. However, you must be cautious and ensure that the quality of the education you are receiving is not only sufficient but excellent, preparing you amply for the new field you are exploring. In addition to taking the traditional courses, there are numerous other ways to learn about a new field or discipline. You should seek mentorship from those in the new field. It is often available through the offices of a scientific or professional society. These societies are usually interested in recruitment to their field so they offer resources to those interested in exploring the discipline. Volunteering a few hours a week will allow you to see a new area firsthand. You will make useful contacts and have opportunities to network and to have people in the field see your work. They may be able to provide references for you down the road. You may also be able to produce some work that could become part of the portfolio that you will present when applying for nonacademic positions.

11.2 LIFE SCIENCES PLATFORM

The training in biomedical or life science research you complete toward your graduate degree will likely become a platform upon which to train and enter a new field. Combining fields or disciplines provides a very compelling set of skills that can foster innovation. This is very attractive to recruiters. For example, financial institutions may seek employees with a strong science background to work with their investment teams.

11.3 JOB CHOICES

In the health care area, you may consider clinical diagnostic fields such as clinical chemistry, clinical microbiology, clinical genetics, and clinical molecular diagnostics. These do not require an MD degree, but do require additional postdoctoral type training and most often certification by a professional body. Many graduate students find that these clinical pathways make very good use of their life sciences research background by providing them with jobs in applied science and health care delivery. There may be a component of research in many of these positions, especially those in academic health science centers.

There are the traditional nonacademic research scientist positions in pharmaceutical and biotechnology industries in which you remain a bench scientist and/or become a laboratory or program manager removed from the bench, but still directing research. Some scientists in these positions maintain close collaborations with academic institutions through teaching and research. If you are carrying out scholarly activity, you may be eligible for a university appointment and participate in teaching and graduate student supervision. The university and industry will need to ensure that the requirements of each partner do not conflict, especially with respect to the training of graduate students. The interface between academia and nonacademia is becoming less rigid, and there is a crossover. The interaction between industry and academia can be productive for both sides.

In the pharmaceutical industry, there are many nonresearch opportunities for life sciences graduates including medical science liaison, regulatory affairs, marketing, account management, risk management, and medical affairs to name some.

There are opportunities to use your biomedical and life sciences training as a platform to enter numerous other nonacademic fields. If you enjoy writing, you may consider science writing or editing/publishing. Graduates may find business and the financial side of science to their liking. Financial analysts with a background in life sciences play an important role in many financial institutions. Science policy is an attractive area for some who are interested in available opportunities in government and nongovernmental science and health care agencies and groups. Teaching science at the high school level is another area you may consider since highly qualified scientists enhance the scholarship of high school life science programs. In high school, you can mentor teenagers interested in careers in life sciences, which is one of the attractions of such a job.

11.4 PLACEMENTS AND INTERNSHIPS

Oftentimes successful job placements or internships in industry as part of your academic training lead to offers of nonacademic employment once you graduate. Create a network for yourself through direct contacts with peers, colleagues, faculty, and staff. Word of mouth and creative use of social media are important contact points and often lead to valuable information about job opportunities. You should consider setting up interviews with folks currently working in areas that you are interested in. These are referred to as "informational interviews" in which you find out from the individual about the characteristics of their job and how their position supports their company's activities. Since these are busy people who are not recruiters but are doing you a favor, keep the interview short and well-focused so your questions are answered. You may ask if you can add this person to your network in order to update them on your activities and ask advice as required.

> You Should Set Up Informational Interviews to Become Well Informed About Career Opportunities

11.5 HEAD HUNTERS

There are several well-known human resources companies that specialize in providing scientific staff and recruiting services to the pharmaceutical and biotechnology industries, to government agencies and institutions, to contract research organizations, and to others requiring life sciences graduates. It is worthwhile learning about these companies, understanding how they place scientists, and familiarizing yourself on who pays for what and what obligations you have to the recruiting company. Read all contracts carefully and seek advice as appropriate.

11.6 ADVANCEMENT IN NONACADEMIC CAREERS

The academic path may be considered more straightforward than the numerous paths available in industry, business, finance, government, scientific agencies, and the numerous other jobs you may find yourself in. The general principles, however, are the same in all settings. Be well informed, seek out reliable mentors, and learn how to create opportunities for yourself within your institution. Learn what is required to move up the ranks. Understand how long you should stay at one position and what additional training you need to move forward. Once you have a track record, you may also look outside your institution, especially if you recognize that there are limited opportunities for advancement at your current industry position.

> Learn How to Advance Your Career and Create Plans to Do So

THE GOLDEN RULES FOR SUCCESS

- Be well informed
- Plan ahead but be ready to alter plans as opportunities appear
- Stay focused but be open to new directions
- Choose supervisors and bosses well
- Choose mentors
- Be well trained and seek advanced degrees. Be innovative and learn to assess risk
- Choose to work on important problems that you are passionate about
- Be well versed in accessing funds to maintain and grow your research program
- Work hard and work smart
- Be ready to handle failure and adversity, be resilient
- Budget your time carefully and set priorities
- Practice research integrity
- Be collegial and be a team player
- Choose your collaborators very carefully
- Network and cultivate relationships in your scientific community
- Be a lifelong learner
- Pay attention to and nurture supportive relationships with family and friends
- Acknowledge and thank those who help you on the way to success
- Have fun and keep a sense of humor about you

Appendix: Questions and Answers on Important Issues

These are topics that I am frequently asked about by students and faculty members:

1. **As a senior high school student, is it advisable to participate in a university organized life science/biomedical research program that provides high school students with a glimpse of research and university life?**

   It is a very useful way to spend your time if you have an interest, and especially a passion, for this field. You will benefit most if you have a sound background in high school biology and science and enter a "pipeline program" that is designed to excite you about further academic training in biomedical/life sciences research. You will be building on what you know and you will get a glimpse of your possible future. If you do not enjoy biology, you will likely find the program boring and a waste of time. Being exposed to life sciences in this type of program may foster your interest especially if you do not yet have any specific career interests. However, if you have other passions, you should follow those. It may be that the same university has programs and opportunities in your own area of interest. I had a very bright high school student attend the laboratory to obtain some hands on experience. However, every lunch hour and even during quiet times in the laboratory he spent his time reading history books. He loved history and was only in the laboratory because a family member suggested he try out science. So if you already have a passion, go for it.

   The best university prep programs provide lectures from faculty researchers and mentored research opportunities in an active research laboratory. They are usually held during the summer months. To gain the most out of the experience you should have a well-focused and supervised project which is doable in the brief time you will be in the laboratory. Expect to work hard. This is not a spectator sport. You will probably work with a senior undergraduate student, a graduate student, or a postdoctoral student. Not all experiments work out, in fact, many do not. However, you will learn something even from failed experiments as well.

You should not only interact with the professor but also with the undergraduate and graduate students in the laboratory who can give you a true picture of what it is like to do research. This experience will allow you to make informed choices about your course of study as you enter the university.

During this time you will learn about: laboratory health and safety, how to keep laboratory records, how to talk about your scientific work with faculty and peers, and how to write simple reports and present your research in an oral or poster presentation to your peers and faculty. In terms of techniques and conceptual knowledge, what you learn depends to a large extent on the research project you carry out.

Even at this stage of your education, begin to explore the traditional academic job opportunities as well as the employment needs and opportunities that are plentiful outside academia. For the motivated student, this type of program organized for senior high school students at the university can definitely be inspiring and help define your career path as you prepare to leave high school and enter college or university.

2. **Is there university help for high school science fairs?**

Yes, however you are best served by identifying a professor who has an interest and expertise in your project. Investigate through your science teachers, websites, and through word of mouth (sibling, older friend, etc.) who at your local university is working in your area of interest. The best form of communication is email. Do not send out mass emails to faculty. Customize your email to a few professors who you think can help. Be polite. Describe the rules of the fair. Provide details of your science so that the professor understands what you want and how much time she will need to devote to your project. Make sure you include the dates between which you will be doing your project. Indicate when the project needs to be finished. Indicate times that you are available. Suggest a possible first meeting if the professor is interested in helping you.

You can prepare a short abstract that has a title and the following sections: background of your project; materials and methods; how you are going to do the project; what you are going to analyze once you do the experiments; and what you are likely to conclude. Here are two abstracts from my own full-length publications to give you an idea of how an abstract is written once the project is completed and ready for publication.

Abstract

Wnt3a/β-catenin increases proliferation in heart valve interstitial cells.

Xu S, Gotlieb AI

BACKGROUND: Valve interstitial cells (VICs), the most prevalent cells in the heart valve, mediate normal valve function and repair in valve injury and disease. The Wnt3a/β-catenin pathway, important for proliferation and endothelial-to-mesenchymal transition in endocardial cushion formation in valve development, is up-regulated in adult valves with calcific aortic stenosis. Therefore, we tested the hypothesis that Wnt3a/β-catenin signaling regulates proliferation in adult VICs.

METHODS: Porcine VICs were treated with 150 ng/ml of exogenous Wnt3a. To measure proliferation, cells were counted on day 4 posttreatment and stained for bromodeoxyuridine (BrdU) at 24 h posttreatment. β-Catenin small interfering RNA (siRNA) was used to knock down β-catenin expression. Apoptosis was measured with terminal deoxynucleotidyl transferase dUTP nick end labeling assay. To assess changes in β-catenin, cells were stained for β-catenin at days 1, 3, 6, and 9 posttreatment. Western blot for β-catenin was performed on whole cell, cytoplasmic, and nuclear extracts at day 4 posttreatment. To measure β-catenin-mediated transcription, TOPFLASH/FOPFLASH reporter assay was performed at 24 h posttreatment.

RESULTS: Wnt3a produced a significant increase in cell number at day 4 posttreatment and in the percentage of BrdU-positive nuclei at 24 h posttreatment. The increase in proliferation was abolished by β-catenin siRNA. Apoptosis was minimal in all conditions. Wnt3a produced progressively greater β-catenin staining as treatment length increased from 1 to 9 days. Wnt3a produced a significant increase in β-catenin protein in both whole cell and nuclear lysates after 4 days of treatment. Wnt3a significantly increased TOPFLASH/FOPFLASH reporter activity after 24 h of treatment.

CONCLUSION: Wnt3a/β-catenin signaling pathway is an important regulator of proliferation in adult VICs.

From Cardiovasc Pathol. 2013. 22: 156-66

Abstract

Cell density regulates in vitro activation of heart valve interstitial cells.

Xu S, Liu AC, Kim H, Gotlieb AI

BACKGROUND: Valve interstitial cells, the most prominent cell type in the heart valve, are activated and express α-smooth muscle actin in valve repair and in diseased valves. We hypothesize that cell density, time in culture, and the establishment of cell-cell contacts may be involved in regulating valve interstitial cell activation in vitro.

METHODS: To study cell density, valve interstitial cells were plated at passages 3 to 5, at a density of 17,000 cells/22 $\times$ 22 mm coverslip, and grown for 1, 2, 4, 7, and 10 days. Valve interstitial cells were stained for α-smooth muscle actin and viewed under confocal microscopy to characterize the intensity of staining. To study time in culture, valve interstitial cells were plated at a 10-fold higher density to achieve similar growth densities over a shorter time period compared with valve interstitial cells plated at low density. α-Smooth muscle actin staining was compared at the same time points between those plated at high and low densities. To confirm valve interstitial cell activation as indicated by α-smooth muscle actin staining, valve interstitial cells were stained for cofilin at days 2, 5, 8, and 14 days postplating. To study the association of transforming growth factor β with valve interstitial cell activation with respect to cell density, valve interstitial cells were stained for α-smooth muscle actin and transforming growth factor β at 2, 4, 6, and 8 days postplating. To study the activation of the transforming growth factor β signaling pathway, valve interstitial cells were stained for pSmad2/3 at days 2, 4, 6, 8, 10, and 12 days postplating. To study cell contacts and activation, subconfluent and confluent cultures of valve interstitial cells were stained for β-catenin, N-cadherin, and α-smooth muscle actin. Also, whole-cell lysates of subconfluent and confluent valve interstitial cell cultures were probed by Western blot analysis for phospho-β-catenin at Ser33/37/Thr41, which is the form of β-catenin targeted for proteosomal degradation.

RESULTS: The percentage of valve interstitial cells with high-intensity α-smooth muscle actin staining decreases significantly between days 1 and 4, and at confluency, most cells show absent or low-intensity staining, regardless of time in culture. Similar results are obtained with cofilin staining. Transforming growth factor β and nuclear pSmad2/3 staining in valve interstitial cells decreases concurrently with valve interstitial cell activation as cell density increases. Examining β-catenin and N-cadherin staining, single valve interstitial cells show no cell-cell contact with strong cytoplasmic staining, with some showing nuclear staining of β-catenin, while confluent monolayers show strong staining of fully established cell-cell contacts, weak cytoplasmic staining, and absent nuclear staining. The presence of cell-cell contacts is associated with a decreased α-smooth muscle actin. The level of phospho-β-catenin at Ser33/37/Thr41 is lower in confluent cultures compared with low-density subconfluent valve interstitial cell cultures.

CONCLUSION: Cell-cell contacts may inhibit valve interstitial cell activation, while absence of cell-cell contacts may contribute to activation.

From Cardiovasc Pathol. 2012. 21: 65-73

If help is offered then you have the responsibility to complete the project and attend any required meetings. If you are going to work in the university laboratory, you need to be instructed on laboratory health and safety and any other laboratory guidelines. You must follow all the laboratory rules. Most likely you will work with a student or staff member who will guide you as you pursue your project.

3. **Should I seek out several research experiences as an undergraduate student or should I stick to one laboratory?**

   The answer to this frequently asked question will depend on why you are doing this in the first place. If your main reason is because research experience is an important prerequisite to securing a graduate position in a very good department, then the type of research is not critically important and you may either stay in one laboratory or move around. What is crucial, however, is how well you perform and strong letters of reference you receive praising your research capabilities.

   However, if you want to begin to seriously explore which research path you wish to pursue in the future, choose the specific projects you wish to be involved in and the labs you want to work in carefully. To achieve the goal during your undergraduate years, it is best to begin the process early in year 1 or 2 so that you have the time to experience the breadth of the field. Please note however that if you take this approach you will be privileging breadth over depth as you will not have time in any one lab to complete in-depth work. If your goals are to test your scientific research capabilities or to discover new knowledge which may lead to a substantial published paper, then several projects for credit and/or summer work all in the same laboratory on the same project will provide you with this high impact opportunity. My colleagues and I have had several students who carried out several projects and participated in mentored research opportunities during the summer in the same laboratory and ended up with excellent content expertise on a given topic and even a first authored publication. This type of productivity makes you a good candidate for a graduate scholarship/studentship. It tells the award committee/awarding agency that you indeed have the ability to go in depth on a research question and produce a first authored paper in a very good to outstanding biological journal.

So you must make up your own mind as to how you want to proceed during your undergraduate years: depth or breath. If I were your supervisor and you demonstrate a passion for life sciences in my undergraduate research program then I would certainly be pleased to give you priority to continue working in my laboratory so that you could perform additional experiments and move your project forward. This additional time will allow you to expand your technical and knowledge base and continue to study the problem in depth.

4. **Extracurricular activities take time. Are they worth it?**

Undergraduate students transition from high school where there is time for extracurricular activities, to college or university where the curriculum is heavier and you have to become a very good manager of your time. Like most students, you will probably manage well and find that the extracurricular activities offer enjoyable social interactions as well as a healthy lifestyle. Student clubs may foster new interests and provide opportunities for exercising people skills, teambuilding, and networking. All these extracurricular opportunities should be considered part of your university education. You should enjoy your university experience and benefit from both its educational and sociocultural opportunities.

Graduate student work can be lonely. You work on your own project and you have to deal with the successes and failures. Progress may be slow, and it may take considerable time before you see positive results and feel that all your hard work is paying off.

Extracurricular activities give you an opportunity to change your focus from the research to yourself and to your community. These activities also provide positive feedback over shorter time spans and help to compensate for the longer time frames needed to achieve success at the laboratory bench. Individual and team sports are frequent favorites. The latter allows you to meet other folks outside your own lab group. The university offers numerous opportunities to participate in a variety of clubs and associations. Students may also participate in student and/or university governance. Departments have undergraduate and graduate student organizations that provide social and academic programs for the benefit of their fellow students. Those involved at the leadership level learn how to work together on a team and how to administer programs and events. I have seen successful student groups put on research days where they organize the scientific and social programs, poster boards, the faculty judges, the refreshments and the invited speakers. This is excellent experience for the students since this is what they will be asked to do as faculty members in the academy or employees in industry. Some of our student groups have organized scientific seminars with invited national and international speakers. They create meeting booklets containing the program and speaker CVs, and much more. These activities are not for "credit" but this leadership experience is invaluable and the sense of satisfaction one derives from a job well done is most gratifying.

Many students also are involved in high school outreach programs, sometimes with less advantaged groups in the community. As an undergraduate or graduate student, you may provide mentorship, and even remediation, especially in science, biology, and mathematics. These programs are very valuable to the community as they expose these younger students to university culture and allow them to consider the possibility of a university education once they successfully graduate high school. Attracting and recruiting underrepresented minorities and those from economically disadvantaged communities is a priority for postsecondary educational institutions. Undergraduate and graduate students are excellent role models and mentors for these high school students.

The trick is balance. Extracurricular activities are to be encouraged and are very useful on a personal and on an educational level. However, they should not take over your life and involve major time commitments that take you away from your course work and research program. Students often discover that finding this balance is a constant struggle. One of my own peers became so heavily involved in successfully filling student leadership roles that he ended up failing a year in his professional program. This is not to be emulated, so balance your time commitments carefully.

How do you know when you have lost your balance? When have you taken on too much responsibility? Students tell me that they know when they suddenly become too busy and feel the pressure of not being able to fulfill either their academic or their extracurricular responsibilities. Being rushed all the time takes the fun out of the activity. One of my students handles this through self-reflection. When she feels the enjoyment dissipating and life stress building up, she steps back and reevaluates the commitments being made to the extracurricular activities and then makes appropriate adjustments.

Institutions do recognize the value of extracurricular activities that benefit fellow students and the community. There are annual departmental/institutional awards that recognize achievement and leadership in these areas. These awards are an important part of a stellar CV that academics and nonacademics recognize when hiring faculty and employees.

5. **Should I go to graduate school directly after my undergraduate program?**

There is no standard answer to this question that fits every student. It depends on your own individual circumstances, so there are a few possible scenarios. As long as your decision is well informed then there is no right or wrong choice.

One scenario that you might find yourself in is that after a challenging undergraduate program you are tired of the academic student grind. You need some time to collect your thoughts, explore new avenues, and see the world around you from a nonstudent viewpoint. You are not motivated to continue your schooling at present. You have not developed a passion for research that drives you to plan to continue your formal education immediately. If this is the case then I advise you to take a break. However, give careful thought to how you can have a productive break time. Your mentors can provide useful guidance. Establish objectives and goals during your break which help and guide you to eventually make a decision as to whether to go to graduate school or not.

Another scenario is that after completing your undergraduate degree, you are in the midst of an exciting academic period. Your undergraduate program has given you a direction for career development and you are passionate about what comes next. In this case, continuing on is a good idea. You will not lose your momentum and you are able to take advantage of what you have done so far to propel yourself forward. For example, you may have already made very good progress on the problem that you have been investigating so that if you continue your work, you will be able to be ahead of the game as you enter graduate school. Continuing on to graduate school immediately makes sense since it maximizes your potential for success. You are passionate about the topic and have shown that you can succeed in this area of biomedical/life sciences research.

Another scenario is that you are indeed passionate and motivated about a biomedical or life sciences area of study but you want to catch your breath. In this case, take some time off but arrange your next step before you do so so that you still maintain your academic contacts and momentum. Try to confirm a position for when you return. Since investigators have to plan ahead as well to fill their complement of graduate student positions, this approach can be attractive to both you and your potential supervisor.

Finally, there is another scenario that is becoming more and more common, the "mature" graduate student. You may have decided to attend graduate school this way in the first place or it may just have happened as your life evolved. You stay out of school for a number of years. After having been in the work force and seen the numerous opportunities out there, you have decided that you are ready to return for a formal graduate education. Especially in biomedical and life sciences, you may have to take some courses before you are eligible to apply for doctoral studies. Scientific knowledge is rapidly expanding so your undergraduate education may need to be updated with current, state of the art knowledge. Since you have been working and bringing in a reasonable salary you are likely accustomed to a certain life style. As a graduate student you will probably be unable to match your previous income. If you plan to work outside of the laboratory to increase your earnings, carefully plan this with your supervisor to make sure that you do not diminish your research experience and productivity. Unless you have other sources of income you likely are going to need to adjust your lifestyle. You will need to "down size." Many mature students do very well. They are motivated and passionate about their work, and their life experience is a valuable asset in working in the laboratory setting and being part of the research team.

6. **Should it be hard to speak frankly to my supervisor?**

As a graduate student, you should be able to comfortably speak to your supervisor about anything related to your course or research work. Your personal life is just that, personal. If issues in your life affect your educational pursuits, then it would be wise for you to share these and discuss the issue, in confidence if you deem that necessary, with your supervisor first. Your supervisor may need to seek advice from others at the university, depending on the issue. Normally your supervisor will ask for your permission to do so. Your supervisor may also feel that he needs to refer you to another individual to give you proper advice. Being transparent and open with your supervisor is an important feature of the student−supervisor relationship.

The hardest issue to deal with is a problem with your supervisor. It is always best to speak directly with your supervisor to try to address the problem. Sometimes it may appear like a major problem when in reality it can be resolved rather simply by making the necessary changes. You may, however, want to consult with your graduate coordinator or one of your mentors to seek advice on how best to communicate directly with your supervisor. These issues should be kept confidential so that you and your supervisor can be more comfortable with each other and conduct an open and frank discussion. Supervisors would much rather have an opportunity to initially deal directly with you without intermediaries. What you do not want to happen is for your supervisor to hear from someone else that you have a problem with him. You may, however, need someone to mediate an issue or dispute you have with your supervisor. The most likely person to do so is the graduate coordinator who can bring a neutral and reasoned perspective to the issue at hand. In terms of the departmental chain of command, if the graduate coordinator is unhelpful or unavailable, in most departments, you would meet with the chair, or perhaps a delegate such as a departmental vice-chair of education.

On the lighter side, students often ask if they should speak to their supervisor about matters of general interest. There is no ironclad rule. It really depends on your supervisor's own personality and interests, how busy he is and whether he actually likes to chat. Some supervisors and, for that matter, some peers in the laboratory, like to separate their work from their personal lives and thus they would not want to share personal experiences with their work mates. This should not affect your workplace interactions and is not a cause for concern. Each laboratory will have its own culture and it is up to you to learn it. Then find a way to fit in and benefit from the social interactions.

7. **What can I do if I realize my supervisor is not the right fit for me?**
   You already took the first step in identifying that you perceive an incompatibility issue that is affecting your graduate work and presumably, your ability to progress. Try to define for yourself what the issue or issues are. Is it the supervisor himself? Is it the laboratory group? Is it the department/institution? These distinctions should be clear in your mind because they will influence how you deal with the situation and what your final goals may be. In your own mind, do you feel that changes can be made in your current laboratory and/or supervision that will improve your situation? If the answer to this question is yes, then how can these changes be made? It is likely that you will have to speak to your supervisor in a frank and open manner, express your concerns, and offer some suggestions about how to ameliorate the situation.

   If an immediate solution is not apparent and you do not wish to discuss the issues with your supervisor, then you have to talk directly to your graduate coordinator. She will be able to provide suggestions some of which may not have occurred to you to resolve the situation. She will present your options if you decide to leave your current supervisor and laboratory. You may also consult with members of your student advisory committee. You, your supervisor and your graduate coordinator should try hard to mediate the concerns and solve the problem.

   Remember that you agreed to work in the laboratory and your supervisor chose you instead of someone else. You have both made a commitment to make this work. If you leave there will be a gap to fill in your research team. Your leaving may incur loss of time, resources, and momentum in the research project that you are working on. Still your progress in your own graduate work is of primary concern, and a change in supervision is required if incompatibility exists that cannot be overcome.

   Whatever the outcome, do not let the situation drag on for weeks. Prioritize dealing with the situation and regaining your forward momentum. Finding a new supervisor may not always be easy or quick. There may not be openings available due to lack of space or inadequate funding. If you change supervisors, you will probably change or at least alter your project as well. If you can continue on with your project that would be ideal; however, this may depend on how far along you are in your research, what type of access you have to your current laboratory and reagents, and the availability of someone else willing and able to supervise you in your current project. Be very clear on how much time you will lose in your program and make sure that student stipends are available for you to complete your degree in a satisfactory manner.

Incompatibility with a supervisor does occur. This is why I stress finding out as much as you can about the laboratory group and the supervisor before you join the laboratory. Since graduate student positions are very competitive, as a student, you may be so grateful to be accepted into a laboratory for your graduate program that you overlook or even worse, disregard warning signs that this faculty member's supervision style will not mesh with your needs and will not inspire you in your research work.

8. **What is my responsibility as a student to maintain research integrity?**
Research integrity refers to conducting, reporting, and publishing research work that is honest and untampered. Fraud, falsification, and/or plagiarism undermine the entire scientific endeavor. Honesty in your research program and in your colleagues' is an essential cornerstone of the biomedical and life sciences research enterprise because each scientific discovery is the building block upon which new discoveries are supposed to be made. Each university/research institute has published policies on research misconduct and you must be familiar with them. Loss of integrity has severe consequences for the perpetrator and results in loss of confidence in science by the public. Penalties for broaching integrity may be imposed by the university or institute, a granting agency, or if a crime has been committed, a court of law. Your laboratory records, including all of the raw data, must be available in an organized fashion so that they can be easily and quickly reviewed. Explanatory notes that you take while conducting the experiments being done must be included since they clarify issues in your protocol, experimental work, and data analysis. So it is your responsibility to behave in a responsible manner and maintain the integrity of your research work.

You also have the responsibility to ensure that colleagues, peers, students, faculty, and laboratory staff also adhere to the codes of behavior for research integrity. If you suspect a problem then it is best to first seek advice from your thesis supervisor or if this is where you suspect an issue may have arisen, from your graduate coordinator. Universities and research institutions have policies and processes in place, which are known to their research community, to deal with any allegations of misconduct in research. These must be followed in consultation with the appropriate university or institutional authorities tasked with dealing with allegations of misconduct. All communication should be handled with strict confidentiality and privacy. You should make sure of your facts. Making frivolous or malicious complaints is also an infraction of the behavior codes and must be avoided. Research integrity is taken seriously by all universities/institutions. It is everyone's duty to maintain research integrity and be vigilant of the integrity of both their own research and that of others.

9. **Is occupational health and safety really important?**
   Knowledge and implementation of occupational health and safety regulations, procedures and protocols is very important for all, including students, faculty, scientific staff, administrators, and secretarial staff. It is the responsibility of the institution to have a comprehensive set of regulations, and to provide opportunities for everybody to learn these regulations so they can follow them. This learning process is open to audit by regulatory agencies, which have oversight over safety in the workplace. This is to ensure that all employees know the rules and follow them. Students and employees must be trained before they begin work and records of this training must be maintained. The institutions usually have the overall liability for workplace safety; however in practice, it is the supervisors and managers who provide day to day oversight and enforcement of the regulations and practices. They need to create a safe work environment throughout the institution, including posting appropriate signage in labs and buildings. Preventing accidents is very important. If an accident should occur, knowing what to do in a quick and efficient manner is essential and may help prevent serious injury or worse.
   Life sciences and biomedical research laboratories have many potential hazards. Each institution provides information and appropriate seminars and/or courses to teach occupational health and

safety. Everyone who works in the laboratory must be well aware of this information. You should be aware of personal protective equipment necessary for lab work, and you should be provided with it and wear it when appropriate. For example, wear laboratory coats, gloves, close toed shoes, and protective goggles or splash visors. They are designed to keep you safe and must be worn whenever appropriate. Understanding when to work in a fume hood, how to use, store, and dispose of hazardous chemicals, and how to dispose of sharp objects is extremely important. There should be no food in the laboratory. You must understand all fire regulations and strictly adhered to them. If you use biohazards or radioactive material, you will need to successfully complete a course to teach you safe handling and storage of these hazards. You will not only learn how to work safely with these agents, but also how to dispose of them safely and deal effectively with any mishaps.

10. **How can email and social media create problems for students?**
You are very familiar with digital communications. They are fast, they have the capacity to reach large numbers of people, and they may exist forever in cyberspace. You need to understand the consequences of using these valuable communication tools inappropriately. You must avoid sending messages and information that puts you in a poor light. Think before you send and do not be impulsive in responding to communications sent to you. Several institutions have guidelines for using digital communication on institutional and company URLs. These must be strictly adhered to.
If you misuse digital communications, at the very least you will offend people. However, the consequences can be far more severe. Serious transgressions can result in your being denied a student position or job or even being dismissed from your current position or employment. The stakes are high so you must be very careful and thoughtful about what you post on social media, both text and images. If a problem arises, consult your supervisor and/or graduate coordinator immediately.
Why am I so adamant about what you write in an email or a social media post? After all, everyone knows that it is just an email or a silly social media post! In the age where public disclosure of private correspondences have destabilized political alliances, and where email hacking led to the firing and resignations of business leaders, celebrities, and politicians for some thoughtless remarks revealed in

illegally hacked private correspondences, the danger of communicating too flippantly in an email or posting a picture that is too silly or risqué on social media are just too great. To a potential supervisor or employer, an inappropriate communication may make them think twice about accepting or hiring you. They may wonder whether you are too impulsive and do not think an issue through before you act. They may wonder whether you are unable to control your anger or rage, or whether you are too quick to be provoked and tend to respond inappropriately. These are not characteristics people look for in a potential graduate student, postdoctoral student or employee. In some cases they show that you do not understand confidentiality and the implication of breaching someone else's privacy, or even your own. They may indicate that you cannot assess which communications are in poor taste and which are not. Just as how you dress for a job interview communicates who you are to a prospective employer, your internet and social media portfolios (which are all too often quite accessible!) may send detrimental messages to your future supervisor or employer.

When using email to communicate in a professional capacity, whether you are a student or a faculty member, keep it short and to the point and do not embellish your communication with jokes or inappropriate comments. These may come to mind as you prepare an email or tweet, but resist the temptation, and if you have typed them, don't be afraid to use the delete button. Remember that emails are not retrievable, so once they are sent, they become part of the record, especially for inquiries, legal matters, and similar processes.

If you need to communicate highly confidential and private information, flag it as such in your email; however, it is best to use the telephone or communicate face-to-face. Sometimes it is hard to reach someone by phone so plan a call when you are both reachable. Remember digital phones may not be very secure. The most effective form of communication is still the face-to-face meeting, especially if you only need to bring a small group together. However, as people get busy, it is often difficult to get everyone around the table to discuss an issue. So you need to set your own priorities on how to handle communications, especially for sensitive issues. Do seek guidance from your supervisor, graduate coordinator, Chair or program director and/or mentor.

If you are on a specific social media provider, carefully read the contract that you sign. Focus on issues around confidentiality, integrity of the digital material sent and received, and retention of the content. When in doubt, check with your institutional IT department to obtain expert advice. They are there to provide consultations on IT matters and keep you and your communications safe.

11. **What if I like both research and clinical medicine?**

What comments do you have about the dual degree program MD-PhD for life sciences research?

Traditionally, students with this dual interest have enrolled in an MD-PhD program: a long period of training combining a medical degree and a PhD in one of the life sciences/biomedical research disciplines. These trainees will go on to careers as physician-scientists who usually devote their professional time to well-funded, independent, and collaborative biomedical research. If you choose this career path, you will be carrying out discovery, translational and/or clinical research in the life sciences/biomedical disciplines for at least 60% of the time and up to 80% of your time. The rest of your time is spent in clinical practice. You will probably work in an Academic Health Sciences Centre, although physician-scientists also make valuable contributions outside of academic medicine, in industry and at government agencies, among other places. As you approach the latter part of your physician-scientist training, you need to explore these nonacademic positions very carefully to see if they provide you with a career that fulfills your own personal research, clinical, and life style goals.

With life sciences/biomedical research training, you bring the curiosity, innovation, and rigor of scientific research into the patient care arena. As a scientist and a physician, you will be able to identify important healthcare problems to study, and you will be able to successfully integrate research findings into patient care. The physician-scientist is very comfortable working on investigations of pathogenesis, prevention, diagnosis, prognosis, and treatment of disease.

As a physician-scientist, you will be well positioned to bridge the gap between basic science and clinical medicine and thus, facilitate the training of medical students, residents, fellows, and your own colleagues. This will enable you to teach state-of-the-art medicine and keep your trainees and colleagues at the forefront of advancing clinical care. Many physician-scientists are able to effectively communicate the excitement and the value of biomedical research to undergraduate and graduate students as well as to the lay public.

Before you embark on training to become a physician-scientist investigate the field carefully. You need to decide whether you have the interest, motivation, and stamina to train to become a physician-scientist. To be successful, this career should fit well with your intellectual interests, with your academic strengths, with your own cultural values, and with the lifestyle you see for yourself in the future. Once you make a decision to move forward, put in the effort required to identify the best program for you to train in and the pathways, including nontraditional ones, that will lead you to become a successful physician-scientist.

There are several different pathways to becoming a physician-scientist in addition to the traditional MD-PhD. Some students enter medical school with a completed doctoral degree in life sciences/biomedical research. During their medical training, they may continue to advance their research as time permits. Other trainees will wait to carry out research training until they do a subspecialty residency and combine this with a formal doctoral degree or simply dedicate protected time to carry out research training under the supervision of a faculty member. In all cases, the physician-scientist must dedicate enough time to research training to enable her to become an independent, funded, biomedical researcher. The best advice I can give to people currently starting on this path is to make sure that they are very well trained, have published high quality innovative research, and are up-to-date in their field of research when they apply for physician-scientist positions in Academic Health Sciences Centers.

12. **Can I move from industry and/or the public sector back into academia?**

No career path is fixed in stone. You can move from academic to public to private sector jobs and back (Fig. A.1). You are not burning your bridges, if you choose academia instead of the private sector, or vice versa; however, there are advantages and disadvantages to moving back and forth. On the positive side, you bring both a different approach to science and new and varied knowledge and technical skills with you. Both your employer and you will be eager to see what new and valuable contributions you can make to this

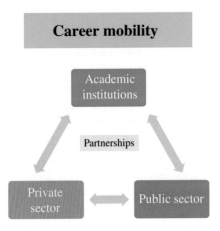

Figure A.1 Career mobility.

new environment, as such variety is a crucial prerequisite for innovation. On the negative side, you may not be entirely comfortable in your new field at first. Being forewarned is being forearmed, knowing that this is a possibility, take the time to fill in any knowledge gaps. As a self-learner looking for new challenges, this should not be too difficult for you.

In moving across the academic–nonacademic divide, you need to be ready and willing to merge the two cultures. They are different, and when you move from one to the other be careful not to remake your new workplace in the image of the one you just left. This is ineffective and, in fact, may be very frustrating and unproductive. Consider blending the two cultures, so that you can synthesize the best of both worlds and develop an improved platform for your work.

Turning scientists into business entrepreneurs has become very fashionable, of late. This process began spontaneously as life scientists made discoveries in their laboratories which they wished to commercialize into products that improve healthcare and benefit the community at large. For those initially involved in this transition, the challenges were daunting since an educational bridge did not readily exist to prepare academic faculty to be both scientists and industrial entrepreneurs. This has changed, as university and research institutes, as well as professional societies, offer courses, programs, and mentoring opportunities to students and young budding entrepreneurs, so that they can develop an understanding and facility with business entrepreneurship. This phenomenon has blurred academic–nonacademic boundaries and working at this interface is increasingly doable and encouraged in many jurisdictions. The concepts and language of intellectual property, business plans, value propositions, networking, and principles of general management are no longer unfamiliar territory for academic scientists.

13. **How do I approach new evolving careers at the interface of disciplines?**
    Careers evolve over time. Established careers are refined and new disciplines arise to meet changing scientific and societal needs either de novo or as branches of an established traditional discipline. These new disciplines spawn new careers. Often folks are not necessarily trained in the new career but instead gradually find themselves working at the interface of two careers and out of necessity fashion a new discipline with all the trappings of a career. You will often hear people say that in the future, even in the near future, we will be working in careers that have not even been thought of or conceived yet. This way of thinking reinforces the notion that students should acquire professional skill sets which are transferable to whatever careers they decide upon. These skills are sometimes referred to as "soft skills" or "professional skills." Included in these are oral and written communication, problem solving, time management, project management principles, self-learning, and networking. These skills are not specific to one career or another. They are universal skill sets that are needed for most careers and should be introduced throughout any life sciences/biomedical research curriculum.

14. **Do I Need to Develop a Fallback Plan (Plan B)?**
    As you develop your career plan, Plan A, you should consider a Plan B (a backup plan) as well. This is both practical and necessary. Both Plan A and B should be compatible with your own interests, goals, strengths, and weaknesses, and should be the outcome of your own self-reflection and the information you have gathered about your career path and destination. Plan A will be your preferred destination; however, internal and external events and circumstances may make it very difficult, or even impossible, to achieve. You should avoid being suddenly thrust into limbo if Plan A does not work out. Do not put "all your eggs in one basket" is the expression that comes to mind. As a well-prepared

student, you should consider several career options at the same time, or at least be open to exploring them, even though your heart is set on one particular career.

For instance, you may have your heart set on medical school, so you put a considerable effort into taking all the prerequisites and building a curriculum vitae that contains curricular and extracurricular experiences which are valued by medical school admission committees. Your focus on medical school may be so extreme that you neglect undergraduate courses that will support other career choices, such as a scientist career in life sciences/biomedical research. If medical school or some other professional healthcare career does not pan out, you are stuck since you have not prepared well for anything else.

Another cautionary tale involves undergraduate students who enroll in life sciences/biomedical thesis-based doctoral MSc or PhD programs to improve their academic record to achieve admission to medical school. What these folks fail to realize is that admission to medical school is still very competitive even with an MSc or PhD. The students still have to achieve an outstanding PhD with excellent course work and high-quality peer-reviewed published papers. Sometimes those who do this find that life sciences research is their true passion and change their career path.

EPILOGUE

My wish is that reading this second edition will provide students, teachers, and mentor(s) with insight and practical tips so that you successfully join the exciting community of researchers and professionals working in the academic, industrial, business, and/or professional realms of biomedicine and life sciences. Understanding the concepts and strategies in this book will provide you with the tools to effectively plan ahead to navigate pathways to achieve a satisfying and successful career.

Your love and passion for biomedical and life sciences is only the first step on a long road. Careful investigation and planning are required to find your calling among the broad array of careers that biological and medical sciences offer. Remember the journey itself should be fun and provide you with a rewarding work-life balance. Well-conceived career development plans at each stage of your training will help turn your interests and passions into concrete options. Keep these plans flexible so that you can take advantage of serendipitous opportunities that arise. With proper mentorship and timely career planning, I trust you will find your niche in the international community of like-minded scientists for whom science is fun, and for whom science fulfills many of their own intellectual, social, and humanitarian needs.

As I conclude this second edition, I urge students and trainees to thank and acknowledge your mentors and supervisors. Do not be hesitant to let your teachers and mentors, among whom I include myself, know how you are doing as you move through your training and into the workforce.

I trust that this book will help you to successfully enter the community of life science and biomedical scholars and practitioners. Whether you continue to carry out research in traditional academic or nonacademic careers, or even in both, or you use your research expertise to enter new hybrid fields, I wish you the very best for a successful and rewarding career.

INDEX

Note: Page numbers followed by "*f*" and "*b*" refer to figures and boxes, respectively.

Printed in the United States
By Bookmasters